PRAISE FOR

This Is
How
I Save
My Life

● ● ● ● ● ● ● ● ● ● ●

"Amy Scher is a brave warrior and a wonderful writer. She is a living example (very much living!) of what it looks like when a woman takes her health, her heart, and her destiny into her own hands. My hope is that this book will inspire many other women to do the same."

—Elizabeth Gilbert,
#1 *New York Times* bestselling author of
Eat, Pray, Love and *Big Magic*

"An *Eat, Pray, Love*–like memoir."

—Pam Grout,
#1 *New York Times* bestselling author of *E-Squared*

"A homecoming of healing, a human story of finding faith, wrapped in a blanket of humor and page-turning candor."

—Kristen Noel,
editor in chief at *Best Self* magazine

"This is the rare book that is both breezy and deep. It speaks to the magic of international travel, and how it can tempt and taunt you to expand into the very best version of yourself, or perhaps become someone entirely new."

—Adam Skolnick,
author of *One Breath* and
over thirty *Lonely Planet* travel guides

"Heartwarming, poignant, and at times deeply funny, this book will shatter the preconceived notions we all subconsciously carry about who we are and what we're capable of."

—Sara DiVello,
bestselling author of
Where in the OM Am I?

"I was drawn to Amy's story immediately. . . . I was rooting for her victory, her recovery, [her] regaining some semblance of a normal life. *This Is How I Save My Life* shows her determination in the faith-invoking journey. Going beyond treatment became something even deeper, something within."

—*San Francisco Book Review*

"In her stunning new memoir . . . the refrain 'we are the healing we've been waiting for' rings throughout . . . a beautiful testament to resilience that veers from the comical to the tragic."

—*Los Angeles Review of Books*

This Is How I Save My Life

SEARCHING THE WORLD FOR A CURE:
A LYME DISEASE MEMOIR

AMY B. SCHER

G

Gallery Books

New York   London   Toronto   Sydney   New Delhi

G

Gallery Books
An Imprint of Simon & Schuster, Inc.
1230 Avenue of the Americas
New York, NY 10020

First Gallery Books trade paperback edition May 2021

This account was previously self-published in different form in 2013 as: *This Is How I Save My Life: A True Story of Embryonic Stem Cells, Indian Adventures, and Ultimate Self-Healing.*

This publication contains the opinions and ideas of its author. It is sold with the understanding that the author and the publisher are not engaged in rendering health services in the book. The reader should consult his or her own medical and health providers as appropriate before adopting any of the suggestions in this book or drawing inferences from it. The author and publisher specifically disclaim all responsibility for any liability, loss or risk, personal or otherwise, which is incurred as a consequence, directly or indirectly, of the use and application of any of the contents of this book.

Some names and identifying characteristics have been changed.

GALLERY BOOKS and colophon are trademarks of Simon & Schuster, Inc.

For information about special discounts for bulk purchases, please contact Simon & Schuster Special Sales at 1-866-506-1949 or business@simonandschuster.com.

The Simon & Schuster Speakers Bureau can bring authors to your live event. For more information or to book an event, contact the Simon & Schuster Speakers Bureau at 1-866-248-3049 or visit our website at www.simonspeakers.com.

Interior design by Bryden Spevak

Manufactured in the United States of America

10 9 8 7 6 5 4 3 2 1

Library of Congress Cataloging-in-Publication Data is available.

ISBN 978-1-5011-6495-8
ISBN 978-1-9821-7726-3 (pbk)
ISBN 978-1-5011-6496-5 (ebook)

For Mom and Dad

Every good bone in my body and bout of inappropriate laughter is because of you. I love you more.
The most.
The end.

None of us is okay and all of us are fine.
—PEMA CHÖDRÖN

AUTHOR'S NOTE

This book is the story of my life based on my own life experiences and memories of them. The dialogue throughout has been re-created from my best recollection of actual conversations. Certain events have been compressed and certain names and characteristics have been changed.

This Is
How
I Save
My Life

1

Guts

DECEMBER 2007

WELCOME TO DELHI, INDIA—IF YOU DON'T
PAY ATTENTION, YOU MIGHT LOSE A LIMB.
A sign with these words is not posted anywhere upon our
arrival, but it should be.

I could have also used a sign that offered GOOD
LUCK! or, equally appropriate, one that read, HAVE
YOU LOST YOUR ACTUAL MIND? In fact, the
signs I need at my first point of entry into the country are
endless.

I am twenty-eight years old when I arrive in magnificent India. I am here with my parents, an updated vaccine
record, and a visa, searching for something I cannot find
at home: *a cure*. In a tiny hospital on the outskirts of Delhi,
a female Indian doctor is offering experimental embryonic

stem cell therapy to patients from all over the world. That is what I have come for.

For the past seven years, my body has been falling apart, sometimes via a slow decline and sometimes like an avalanche. It has been my full-time job to try, mostly unsuccessfully, to put it back together.

My medical diagnoses seem too many to fit in my petite, five-foot frame: inflammation of the heart, autoimmune thyroid disease, brain lesions, chronic fatigue syndrome, encephalopathy, arthritis, chronic inflammatory demyelinating polyneuropathy, fibromyalgia, hypotension, adrenal fatigue, connective tissue disease, leukopenia and neutropenia, endometriosis, and, finally, the reason for them all: late-stage Lyme disease.

But the formal names assigned to my suffering do not begin to convey the actual experience of it. Over the years, there have been hundreds of symptoms, some visiting for only days at a time and others making a permanent home in my body. Each of the symptoms has had a part in destroying not only my physical self but the rest of me as well: fierce, full-fledged body aches making it difficult to move and unbearable to stay still; exposed nerves in my limbs firing with pain and no rhythmic pattern to warn when the worst would come; extreme upper body weakness that kept me from lifting my arms above my shoulders; bottomless fatigue so heavy it was too much effort to move my lips and speak; dangerously low blood counts forcing my immunologist's insistence that I not leave the house; unexplained night sweats that drenched my bedding; cognitive impairment causing me to jumble my words; joints so painful and swollen that lowering myself to the toilet or rolling over in bed put too much pressure on my hips, and was impossible to do alone; light and sound sensitivity that made me afraid of the world; unrelenting headaches that drill through every space in my skull; bouts of labored breathing that had me gasping for air to take just ten steps; patches of skin so sensitive that it felt as if I were being dragged across asphalt naked; and debilitating, painful menstrual cycles triggering dangerously heavy bleeding. No organ or system of my being has been spared.

The intensity of my symptoms has ebbed and flowed, altered by slight relief from treatments and sometimes inflamed by them. They have risen and fallen as tides, knocking me over and stealing my breath, or sometimes, in their gentle mercy, lapping against me with only mediocre force. But always their presence is an undertow; a more subdued reminder that it is never safe to take my eyes off the unsteady shore, off my defenseless body.

I am missing a chunk of my left thigh from a muscle biopsy taken to study my nerves, have faithfully swallowed forty-four pills every day, have listened to the sound of doctors chiseling through my bone marrow to look for clues, have seen all the best experts at the top institutions in the United States—from the Mayo Clinic in Minnesota to Northwestern in Chicago to the University of Southern California, and beyond—hearing the dreaded words over and over: "We don't know how to fix you."

I have suffered through experimental IV medications, rigorous physical therapy, almost a hundred hyperbaric oxygen treatments, self-administered daily antibiotic injections, countless medications, far-reaching alternative approaches, and life-threatening side effects worse than the original symptoms. Doctors often refer to me as *a mystery*.

By the time I land at Indira Gandhi International Airport in India, for what I believe is the very last thing on the very last list of things to try, I am thankful to be a bettered version of who I once was, during my worst days on this earth. Just two years before, I was mostly bedridden with pain in every inch of my body, in a semicomatose state from heavy-duty medications, and dependent on near-constant care by others.

In my somewhat rehabilitated stage, I feel a little bit repaired, like the first time after an epic cold when you are grateful just to breathe from at least half of one nostril again. I try to be thankful for what I do have. I can function at the most basic level of taking a shower and leaving the house, but I haven't been able to work in years. My life is small and square. Still, I *am* living. In order to do so, I need a constant barrage of narcotic medications, nerve stabilizers, and anti-anxiety medications to try to control the symptoms that remain: excruciating systemic nerve pain, paralyzing fatigue, a broken immune system, heart complications, and the weight of an illness that feels heavier than my whole body. I have perfected the dosing and rotation of my prescription medications as a temporary way to experience a fragmented life—even, at times, a joyous one. I try to convince myself that where I am now is "good enough." I keep my eyes glued on the bright side: that I am walking, talking, and driving again; that I live on my own; and that, even though things are not perfect, I am better than where I've been before. But the real truth is that I'm still a mother-freakin' mess. Although looking at me, you might not know anything has ever been or is still so seriously wrong. I style my wild, curly hair every single day, I paint on my makeup, and I fake being seminormal in the very best way I can.

Inside the places that no one knows but me, my heart is split in a million pieces because I am a human being who is lodged in the in-between—in between living and dying. I want to be better than "good enough." If I don't move the goalposts for my own life, who will? I want not only to stay alive, but to *be* alive, to lead a life. I am more afraid of living in this condition forever than I am of dying from it.

I am also alone—partner-less—for the first time in eight years. I am struggling to adjust to life without Jay, the man who took care of me, but also to whom I carelessly gave away all of myself.

Because of all this, I am here in India. I am ready to let everything go and trade it for a life. I am here to get the cure. I am also here to gather the things I have no idea I need, but that is totally unknown to me at this moment. I am here, maybe somewhat irresponsibly, to risk my own life to find it.

It was only three months earlier, as I inhaled the sweet smell of sugarcane in Maui, that I first heard about this highly controversial treatment, which might give me the life I was looking for.

I had just finished a grueling Lyme disease treatment in Chico, California, a small Northern California college town dripping with greenery and hippies. That's when my parents sat me down on my brown tweed rented couch, next to my rented TV in my newly rented apartment. After I'd left Jay and, with him, almost everything I owned, nothing in my life was mine anymore.

"It would be good for you to do some writing," they said with both joy and hesitance, revealing a brochure from a writers conference on Maui. But I think what they might really have been saying was: *This is no life for you. We don't know if you'll ever have one. You want to write a book. Go do the only thing that hasn't been taken from you: your writing.* "And we might have already signed you up!" they jumped to tell me, preempting my *no way* (which was exactly what

I planned to say). I tried to reject the generous offer, re-minding them it was a good day for me if I made it out of the house or just to the kitchen to make my own food, and that I hadn't written a single thing in forever anyway. But I stared a few seconds too long into their hopeful eyes, and succumbed to the superpower of Parental Jewish Guilt.

That's how I ended up on the lush island of Maui, where I met Amanda, a paraplegic who had just returned from a stem cell clinic in India after being treated for a spinal cord injury. Each of us having arrived at one of the conference sessions at the completely wrong time, we started chatting, at first mostly about how we both managed to screw up our schedules so perfectly in sync.

"I made my way here straight from India after receiv-ing stem cells!" she explained in her singsongy Australian accent. "Look, I can wiggle my toes! Isn't that wild? Eight weeks ago, I couldn't move anything from here down." She pointed to her belly button. We immediately bonded over our commonality: our struggling bodies and our desperate desire to heal them. "Ah! The doctor who treated me in India knows about Lyme disease. You should contact Dr. Shroff. Go get stem cells, maybe!" She said it like it was a casual suggestion for dessert. *Go get cheesecake! And maybe get it with strawberries!*

There was much that came during the short months between serendipitously meeting Amanda and the day

I booked my flight to Delhi. First, the doubts: Maybe I really wasn't sick enough for *this*? Amanda couldn't walk. *That* was serious enough for an experimental treatment in India. Could I even survive a twenty-one-hour flight? Where was I going to find the $30,000 for treatment? Who would go with me? What if it was a scam? And OMG, again, where was I going to get $30,000?

When I got home from the conference and told my parents every thought in my brain, they said only two things: "We'll figure out a way," and, "If you're going, we're going too." So I contacted Dr. Shroff, organized and sent my medical records, waited for the "Yes! You can come!," started fund-raising, and had the Indian visas rushed (my first lesson about India: all things can be expedited for the right price). The only thing left to do after all that was totally ignore any practical rationale that told me I was absolutely and completely insane for doing this.

As I said, there was a lot that happened to get me to India—but compared to what felt like the weight of a thousand pounds I'd carried up to that point, the decision to go was a feather.

I *needed* India. I felt this truth in my bones. India might be my exotic healing miracle, my saving grace, the country that delivered me my long-awaited alternate destiny: health. After all I had been through, I believed I was truly ready.

I am a Virgo to the core—a logic-loving, process-of-elimination, pragmatic decision maker. These traits mean that I don't make decisions quickly or gracefully. I've been known to agonize over where to go to dinner like it's my last meal on earth, read hours of online reviews for something that costs five dollars, and obsess over which color to get my toes painted at the salon, even though I always choose an optimistic shade of blue, and it chips off in a week anyway. But for this, the most important decision of my twenty-eight-year-old life, I didn't make lists of pros and cons or even give any decent consideration to what it might actually be like when I got there—easy, difficult, or epically scary. I only set my mind on a singular mission: *to go get the cure in India so I could come home and get on with the rest of my life*. This was *Life or Death*, not *Eat, Pray, Love*. There would be no epic spiritual crisis to endure, no humorous travel tales to tell, and there was zero chance of falling madly in love.

I couldn't hear the Universe laughing in my face back then, but I am sure now that it was.

In reality, nothing could have readied me for what was to come, because India is not just another destination to prepare for, like Thailand, Mexico, Costa Rica, and all those I had visited before it. India is different. India is its own world. India is not for the faint of heart or for the takers. You do not go to India for what you want and carry it away with ease. But I had no idea about any of that. I had a blinding naïveté about what was about to happen to me, which in hindsight was possibly a very good thing. As I arrive at the Delhi airport, I am completely unable to foresee how fiercely India is about to shake me.

With what seems like no effort at all, I am being launched over broken floor tiles via a wooden wheelchair that is tilted thirty-five degrees to the left. My blond hair and white skin are calling attention to me. Mom and Dad are running behind us, desperately trying to keep up. People are pointing and staring at us as I attempt to deflect the discomfort of being a foreign sight. My own thoughts are quickly drowned out by the deafening buzz of Hindi chatter.

I have no time to process the enormity of it all as my wheelchair escort, whose name I don't know, maneuvers me through my new world without caution. While I can walk somewhat confidently on level pavement now, when the ground is rough or I have to walk a decent distance, I use a wheelchair. My own legs are more stable than this wobbly wheelchair, though, and that's not saying much. It has one rickety wheel and is missing its foot pegs. My ride has to be continually corrected and realigned in order to stay on course. When my wheelchair escort isn't paying full attention, we veer into other passengers who are forcing their way outside.

This unpredictable ride mirrors this life of mine, in

which I always feel about three seconds away from being dumped right out onto the floor, left to struggle back up again while everyone else flies past me with ease.

When we exit the double doors of the airport baggage claim into the great wide open and I see my new world for the very first time—tattered, worn, tired, dirty, and clouded in debris—I see myself.

Everything in me comes to a screeching halt.

This is where that sign should go. WELCOME TO DELHI, INDIA—IF YOU DON'T PAY ATTEN-TION, YOU MIGHT LOSE A LIMB.

I am smacked by an assault on my senses. There is a blast of different noises coming from every single direc-tion: construction equipment, loudspeaker announcements in multiple languages, and boisterous laughing. I see a man standing in the middle of the sidewalk singing loudly to himself. A cloud of smoke rushes toward me, but I can't figure out where it's coming from. My throat stings on contact. On the other side of the street, I see a huge park-ing lot. Most of the cars in it are white and Toyota-looking in size and style. I have no idea how people tell them apart when they come back to the lot. The asphalt of this park-ing area is buckled, with large parts completely missing, exposing patches of dirt that sit a full ankle-twist below street level. The night air is thick with a gray haze, but I don't see a fire. People are yelling, and I can't tell if they are angry at each other or screaming into the Universe just to be heard. It is total and utter chaos.

This is when I realize we have lost my parents. I can't locate them anywhere in the sea of people. Trust me, if they were here, I'd spot them. You couldn't miss two New York natives in this crowd if you tried.

My mom, Ellen, is two parts badass and one part stereotypical Jewish mother. She wears the pants in our family. But if you know a Jewish mother, you knew that already. She is full of love and funny as hell, and does everything in life with a determined-to-kick-some-ass stride. She walks fast and talks even faster with her thick Brooklyn accent. When a song from *Dirty Dancing* comes on, she can't help but break out her moves as her blond ponytail swings along. When I was growing up, my mom and her best friend owned a boutique chocolate store. In the back corner of the store was a secret closet filled with their best seller: X-rated chocolates. Sometimes I'd come home from school and she'd be in the kitchen humming "Hungry Eyes" while pouring chocolate into nipple candy molds. *This* is my mother.

My dad, Abraham Solomon Scher, came into this world with a big name, a big weight (thirteen pounds), and a spirit to match them both. This bald, bearded Santa Claus lookalike tells the best Woodstock stories you'll ever hear and has either wise advice or a wiseass joke for every crisis you might endure. He is obsessed with breaking and then fixing things, the super powers of Velcro, and befriending every stranger he meets. He often wears a red clown nose just to make people smile. When my younger brother, David; my older sister, Lauren; and I were growing up, Dad privately told each of us that we were his "favorite." He'd whisper it in our ears, write it in cards, and sneak it into conversation whenever he could. Then he always added his P.S. *Don't tell the other kids!*

My mom and dad are my very best friends.

Parked on the curb, without my parents, I am staring at the parking lot in total overwhelm. I have felt like a lost soul for quite some time, but feeling like a lost child is worse. Tears burn my tired eyes.

What seems like a decade later, but is probably only a minute, Mom and Dad appear out of nowhere with an upbeat young man holding a sign that says our last name, SCHER. He is in his early twenties with unblemished, milky cocoa skin. His teeth are so white that he must bleach them every morning and night.

"My name is O.P.!" he belts out with a huge grin. "I am here from hospital Nutech Mediworld to gather you, Mom, and Dad!"

My parents are smiling at their new hero.

Two men who are dragging our luggage accompany

him with four suitcases for the three of us for eight weeks. O.P.'s wide and dazzling smile makes him look eager with his every word.

"The hospital has sent me to pick you up!" he says, motioning to me with a wink and a nod. He flips his perfectly parted thick mound of dark hair and we follow him.

O.P., our new leader, is speaking in Hindi to his team, laughing as he tips his head from side to side. He is a wave of joy. Weaving and dodging with no effort at all, he maneuvers us through hundreds of cars.

I watch with anticipation as Mom and Dad try to process and react to the shock of their disordered new surroundings. This is their first time out of the United States. They didn't even have passports before I brought them here, on this grand undertaking, to this beautiful, messy, wild country. Back in 1976, they traveled across the country from New Jersey in a brown VW bus they named Bernie, and settled in California to start a family. This is pretty much the extent of their travels, up until this moment. What have I done to them, my sweet parents, who have come to the ends of the earth for me?

O.P. halts and turns to address us. "Now!" he announces with gusto. "You"—he points to the three of us—"will go in thiiis car!" He pauses. "Aaaaand . . . your bags"—he points—"will go in thaaaat car."

My mind is blank. *Whaaaat?* I can't make any words go

to my lips to respond, but am not sure what to say anyway. He wants us to part from our belongings. He is sporting an extra-extra-huge smile, to assure us that his plan is a sound one. In front of us are two white minivans, but far less superior in size to those we see in the States. They are something like *mini* minivans. Everyone knows not to go with unknown men in unmarked white vans, especially without any of your stuff. And while I certainly know better, I somehow completely trust him.

I make eye contact with my parents in an effort to have a nonverbal conversation that brings some clarity about what we should do here. I can hardly think straight, between my narcotic painkillers, antianxiety meds, no sleep, and it being first thing in the morning California time. I half-smile toward Mom, asking with my face, *Do you think this is okay?* She turns her eyes away and stiffens her body. Read: *What did you get us into?* When I look at my dad, he is clenching the travel pouch holding his all-important documents that is dangling around his neck. He has a look of sheer terror in his eyes, his rosy, plump cheeks glowing. I think he is planning to tie himself to his luggage to make sure it goes with us.

O.P.'s face is frozen in sheer delight, as if he's about to hear wonderful news in response to his proposal.

"Let's go then?!" he questions excitedly. In the quick second that I look away to privately contemplate, I spot an Indian man's leg become pegged under a moving car and his army-green luggage flies from his cart and hits the gravel. The white four-door car stops and reverses slightly, the victim's leg is released, and no one seems to care. He gathers his dust-covered bags from the ground and limps away, waving his hand at no one.

I realize I need to make an executive family decision about this luggage, because although I am the child, I feel like the parent at this moment. They are here because of me. I owe them at least the appearance of bravery. But I am terrified.

I was thirty thousand feet in the air on the plane here, fourteen hours into our twenty-one-hour journey, when I experienced my first real moment of massive doubt about this whole thing. The plane, and my destiny, were already well in flight.

It all started with having to pee. I unbuckled my seat belt and shimmied down the aisle to the bathroom. I didn't have far to go because I was only three rows away from it—the worst possible section to be in on an international flight. I kept my sweatshirt hood pulled loosely over my head, feeling a false sense of privacy. I was fourth in line among my fellow full-bladdered passengers. But the thing about this line was that there was no actual formation. Two beautiful Indian women draped in saris plus one Indian businessman in dress pants and a half-untucked shirt were gathered in the short galley way, arranged in no particular fashion. When I joined the congregation, they moved closely toward me, their eyes fixated on my face, their clothes kissing mine.

I read many travel books before leaving home, all of them touching upon the cultural differences between India and America in some way. Personal space, as they all described it, was not as important in Indian culture. This was the first time I experienced this truth for myself, but it most certainly wouldn't be the last. One by one, the Indian passengers drew in around me, and soon five people were questioning why I was on this flight.

"I'm going for medical treatment that I can't get in America," I said, giving minimal details. "The nerves in my legs are damaged and it's very painful."

I had lost the energy to explain my condition in its entirety. Lyme disease can be complicated to understand and, especially in its chronic form, difficult to cure. It is caused by the bacterium *Borrelia burgdorferi*, which is most commonly transferred by certain types of ticks and, some believe, by mosquitoes, flies, and fleas. If the infection is caught early on, it may require only a short dose of antibiotic therapy. However, like me, the majority of people never find the tiny tick that bit them, see the bite itself, or get the bull's-eye rash that's commonly associated with Lyme. When this happens, and the infection goes undi-

agnosed and untreated, it can become incredibly dangerous, especially for those with weakened immune systems.
The bacteria can attack the immune system, burrow in the
bone marrow, hide and evade treatment, and destroy multiple body systems. This is called chronic, or late-stage,
Lyme disease. That's where I am.

But to this audience on the plane, I left it at the legs.

"Oh! You are so brave. It's a rough city." The flight at-
tendant clapped nervously. "Actually, my mother had very
bad leg pain. She drank tonic water and it was a success!"
I giggled silently in my mind. *Ahhh, if only tonic water
really did the trick.* But then I thought, *Wait—did I try that?*
Tonic water cost seventy-five cents, and I was on my way
to a "rough city" for a $30,000 medical experiment in the
most vulnerable state of my life.

This talk of tonic water triggered one of my greatest fears:
that there is something silly and uncomplicated that I've
missed—the elusive, unturned stone. I have heard stories
about Lyme disease patients who struggled for years, and
then found a straightforward missing piece—something
like vitamin B_{12} shots, a detox supplement, juicing, or an
additional antibiotic to add to their regimen. It did the trick
and then they were on their merry way to healing! Just like
that. These are the stories that haunt me; driving me back
again and again to the thought of *What am I missing?* It is
this simple question that stalks my every move, doubling its

force and persistence when I try to resist it. Why can't my thankless body take one of the hundreds of things I've offered it and actually use it? But at this point, it's been pretty well confirmed that that's not going to happen.

In fact, it was only the year before this trip that I turned my life into *Mission: Try-Everything*. Because you just never know. The first thing I ever tried, the Carrot Juice Cure, caused my hands to turn orange from a beta-carotene overdose. All that juicing was colorful but not very effective. I then moved on to drinking cow colostrum via the brags of an online group swearing the early secretion of bovine breast milk was a miracle. One word for that experience: *gross*. I also saw various psychics and intuitives who gave me vague information like "It seems your legs don't work" (thank you!) or offered cryptic messages such as "Your body is full of toxic oil!" (what?) and "You have a terrible relationship with your mother, yes?" (um, no). At one point, I had a session with a healer, whose specialty I never really figured out, who swirled his hands over me and talked to my body in a gibberish language. He seemed as broken and confused as I was. To this day, I still love all things metaphysical—intuitives, mediums, healers, astrologers, crystals, angel communicators, and palm readers—but it's pretty clear that at that time I did not gravitate toward the most talented guidance out there. There was also the Master Cleanse (a.k.a. the Lemonade Diet), which has been around since the 1940s. For twelve days straight, I would drink lemonade only: homemade with cayenne pepper and agave. But several days in, I choked from accidentally sniffing cayenne pepper up my nose and called it quits.

After all that, it seemed stupid to *not* try the tonic water. Because, well, *what if?* That tonic water might be *it*.

On the next beverage round, I asked for a glass of it. I drank it with my fingers crossed, a superstition from childhood I still sometimes honor in times of great need. I waited. It did nothing. I still had electrocuting pains in my legs and felt exhausted as if I were a million years old. I hated to be relieved by this, but to find a cure on my way to India would seriously suck.

That is why, when I see my mom's face in that ramshackle Delhi airport parking lot, blatantly unsure about our next move with O.P. and the white vans, I force my bravery. I am fueled by the confidence that I even tried *one last thing* (again!) on the way here. Whatever happens from here on out needs to happen. I commit to this for the foreseeable future and decide not to look back.

"Let's go!" I tell O.P., confirming that we will indeed part with our luggage in a foreign land, at night—based on the promise of a man we met ten minutes ago, because he acted like it would be totally fine. I have not had any luck with prayers so far, but I close my eyes and say a short one for kicks: *Dear Universe, please help make sure that our luggage meets us at our destination. Thank you and amen!* If Nutech Mediworld hospital embraces the arrival of both my family *and* all our luggage tonight, I will consider it a miracle.

Mom and Dad cannot pile into the van fast enough. Once O.P. closes the door to seal out the chaos, we all collectively exhale, forcefully enough to signal cautiously optimistic relief.

"Shit," my dad says with a laugh, breaking the silence, his big lovely belly jiggling like it does when he's thoroughly entertained. Mom and I laugh too, because from the assumed safety of inside this van, things actually start to seem pretty funny.

O.P. acts as a tour guide, talking on and off for the entire bumpy ride into the night. He turns around from the front seat often, taking his eyes off the road. "So, here you are!" he declares. "You like India?" *So far I only like it because I have survived it*, I think. "Yep!" my mom chimes in, the perfect student, or maybe just startled with fear. The half hour of rough and rugged driving thrashes my digestive system and rattles my nerves. The van bounding over the uneven street sounds like falling rocks. We are thrusting in and out of traffic (how is there such terrible traffic at ten o'clock at night?), and the noise of honking horns is so constant that, after a while, it's just a background roar.

"We're here!" O.P. exclaims as we stop without slowing down first. We are outside a modern-looking three-story building faced with mostly tinted windows. I tilt my head to look up from inside the van. Directly behind us, van number two arrives, canceling the possibility that we'll be dubbed the idiots who let strangers steal our belongings. At least, not tonight.

Climbing out of the mini minivan and into the mildly cool winter air, I hear at least fifty dogs wailing. Horns are angry and ambitious. People are walking and shouting to each other across the busy street. The sky is dark, but the entire city is high with energy. The smell of a fire has followed us.

This twenty-bed facility in South Delhi, squished between a small hotel and a bank with an armed guard stationed outside, will be my new home. The hospital's entrance has a wheelchair ramp alongside the stairs, which we make our way up. We are greeted at the doorway by a group of smiling staff. It feels like we've arrived at Disneyland for a special event. The hospital, humble in appearance, looks clean, smells neutral, and is actually nicer than I had envisioned. The chairs in the lobby area are wooden and clunky, like those you might see in a doctor's office where the furniture hasn't been replaced since the seventies. The royal-blue cushions paired with the wooden frames offer an almost exotic, resort-style feel. The floors are shiny, freshly mopped and maybe waxed.

"Miss Amy?" one of the young women questions, edging toward me in a shuffle. She is dressed in a pressed white nurse's outfit, her hair pulled back in a perfect bun. She is petite, with a tone that is quiet and kind.

"That's me," I respond, raising my hand just to be clear. All the other nurses, who are about her same small size and look to be in their twenties, are grouped around her just watching.

"I am Sahana," the nurse says. I am bad with names and usually forget before the person is even done telling me. I focus hard and review in my head where I am so far: *O.P. Sahana*. Two is easy. "Ready for your room? We show you now."

Mom and Dad are staying at a small bed-and-breakfast a few blocks away for the six weeks they are here with me. For the final two weeks of my treatment, I'll be in Delhi by myself. This plan seemed fine when we made it at home, but I am, all of a sudden, nervous about it now.

"Can I take you to your new place?!" O.P. asks them, putting his hand out to offer them a lift. We wrap our arms around each other for a lingering hug, and they are gone.

Sahana and her gang of "sisters" (*sisters* is the term for nurses in India) lead me to the elevator, which delivers us to the second floor. Two, my lucky number. Well, twenty-two is actually my lucky number, because two twos are obviously better than one. But I take two when I need it most. Now, I need it most.

Through the walls in the corridor leading to my room I can hear patients watching TV. A few are mingling in their doorways and stop to smile. Sisters bustle about, walking around with blood pressure cuffs that are reminiscent of another era.

When we get to the end of the hall, Sahana points to the left corner room: my new home for the next two months. I enter, the girls following and observing my every move closely. As it turns out, my new home is a pleasant surprise. I take a quick inventory of the space. My room is decorated in bold blues; the walls match the chair cushions downstairs and the sheets are a more subtle shade. A plasma TV is affixed to the wall. Score! I have wired Internet—it will be slow, but definitely better than none. Email has been the only consistent lifeline to the world these past years, and I don't want to lose it now. The hospital bed is smaller than my bed at home, but after sitting up in a plane seat for so long, it's as good as a king-size at a luxury hotel. There is a small royal-blue fold-out mattress pad next to it that converts into a chair for extra seating. I have a million different lighting options, although when I flick them on and off, none of the switches correspond correctly to the closest bulbs. In the corner of my room, there is a mini refrigerator. On it are a loaf of bread labeled "brown," Indian crackers, cereal, and bananas. There is a stack of sunflower-yellow-colored bowls, two forks, two spoons, and a knife.

Next to it is an electric teakettle, more modern than the old-school stovetop teapot I have at home. Inside the fridge I find a box of milk labeled "soya." At home, I eat mostly organic. Here, I don't recognize the brands and can't read the ingredients. It's probably for the best.

After I inspect my room in its entirety, I go straight to the large window over the bed and peek out from behind the thick blue fabric roll-up blinds. From here, I have a perfect view of the wide-open main street. I see a monkey on the roof directly across from me chasing and jumping around for trash that is blowing about in the wind.

Stepping cautiously into the square bathroom, I am shocked into new territory. I'm immediately confused by the shower because it has no door, curtain, or lip. The floor of the shower is the same floor that extends to the rest of the bathroom. The toilet sits right next to this shower and the drain for the whole bathroom is in the middle of the floor. It reminds me of an outdoor beach shower that you have to wear flip-flops in, but this has the added awkwardness of the toilet. I can't imagine how I'd use this without getting the entire bathroom soaking wet.

"It is not like your home?" one of the girls asks, perplexed by the amount of time I spend staring.

I smile and sit on the toilet to demonstrate. From this position, I reach over a few feet and playfully grab the detachable showerhead, holding it over my head. "You see, at home, I couldn't pee and wash my hair at the same time." They look horrified, as if this is something I will actually do now that I've discovered it. "Very different," I say. I privately rename this combination the "shoilet," because it's a little bit of a shower and toilet sharing the same space.

"Rest. You need sleep," Sahana instructs, now that our bathroom lesson is over. I nod. "Tomorrow, nine a.m., you go downstairs. You will meet Dr. Shroff. We will ring Mom and Dad." I know I desperately need sleep, but there are so many questions: When will my treatments start? What will the protocol be? Did my parents even make it to their hotel? And, oh crap, if they didn't, how would I ever even know?

When the caravan of sisters leaves, I am alone for the very first time in this unfamiliar world. Everything feels still and I am surprisingly at ease, except I can't seem to ignore the strong smoke odor permeating my room. I begin to investigate for a short circuit somewhere along a wall. In my early twenties, I worked at a newspaper in the editorial department, and even though it's almost a decade later, experiences in my life still sometimes cause story headlines to involuntarily flash in my head. Right now, it is: *Girl Tries to Beat Incurable Illness, Perishes in Hospital Fire.*

After no defect is found inside, I look outside once again. I see a barrel full of smoke, but no fire. It seems several men across the street are huddling over their burned-out bonfire to stay warm. The smell of the outside world is leaking in through my unsealed concrete walls. Looking more carefully, I can see light through the cracks where the corners meet and spaces where the windows don't quite match up.

Climbing onto my bed, I sit erect, completely motionless for a minute, trying to fasten myself into my new reality.

I am not sure what to do with my first empty moments here, worried that if I stop for too long to think, I will be afraid. I feel like I should be freaking out, but I am somehow okay. I feel like being somewhere new gives me something new. Refreshed optimism, perhaps. Or maybe it will ultimately be only a distraction from the inevitable—that I can't be cured.

The wailing from the dogs outside begins to grow louder and then retreats. I finally dig my crumpled pajamas from my suitcase and huddle in the bathroom to change, not confident that my room is totally private from the outside world. The morning is soon approaching, and if this bed feels as uncomfortable to sleep in as it is to sit on, it might come much too soon.

Unpacking my medications, I quickly cover the night table next to my bed. I can only fit on it some of what I need to tend to my high-maintenance body. I have various kinds of oral antibiotics that I take for the Lyme disease.

I have a whole set of medications for the coinfections—additional infections from ticks that often come along with Lyme disease. I have good-bacteria probiotic pills to try to cancel out damage from the antibiotics, and supplements that help my liver detox. I have gallbladder pills to prevent gallstones—a side effect of one of the drugs. I have antacids to offset the gallbladder medication and a special drink to help flush my kidneys. I have horse-pill-sized vitamins for when I can't eat. I have needles, syringes, and vials of antibiotic powder that need to be mixed with lidocaine for my injectables. All of this, to try to stay ahead of the Lyme disease and its symptoms, is a process reminiscent of the Whac-A-Mole game of my youth. As soon as I smack down one pop-up monster infection, virus, set of symptoms, or endangered organ, another appears out of nowhere. This is my life, a constant monster-smacking mess—so confusing and exhausting that I have spreadsheets to help me keep track of symptoms, dates, and intensity so I can accurately relay everything to my doctors. I think it's pretty clear that the monsters have the upper hand.

As I sit on the bed in a cross-legged position and ten thousand miles away from home, with everything at stake, the feeling I had when I made the decision to come here returns to me. I *need* India. I still feel this truth in my bones. But all the reasons I think I need India will turn out not to be any kind of truth at all. India, with all its guts and glory, will take me, overtake me, undertake me, and painstakingly spit me out. It turns out that India will also love me, care for me, and cradle me in ways so magnificent it will be worth every mile.

2

Holy Cow

WEEK ONE

"Wait till you go out there, baby," my dad says, out of breath, eyes full of sheer amazement.

My parents have just walked the two blocks from their hotel right off the busy main drag, and into the safety of the hospital lobby. Daylight has brought not only them to me, but the blank page of the first day in my new world.

"Oh boy!" my mom follows cheerfully. "I'm shvitzing from crossing that main road! It's nuts!" Despite it being the Indian winter now, an average of about fifty degrees Fahrenheit, she is indeed sweating. In one sentence, my mom has brought New York to India.

The hospital is located in Green Park, sometimes referred to as the lungs of Delhi, because it is near one of the largest green areas in the city. But I see nothing green here. While Green Park was described to me as a posh area of the city, it so far feels more like an area of LA that tourists are warned to stay away from. There is trash every single place I look. Instead of there being bins, garbage is piled up on the curbs—except there isn't even really a curb. From my own wide gaze out the giant glass windows, which reach from top to bottom at the front of the building, I can see why Mom and Dad are so discombobulated. It's a perfect view into total disarray. A cow is stopped in the middle of the road and halting traffic; people are stuck in the three-wheeled taxis known as *tuk-tuks* waiting for the cow to move; families of four are stacked on motorcycles whizzing by the tuk-tuks; groups of men use brooms to sweep up tornadoes of dirt caused by the motorcycles; and a monkey in a dress is running in the center divider alarmed by it all. Yes, a monkey. In a dress. We're definitely not in La La land anymore.

Inside the lobby, there is loud buzzing and chattering that you'd expect from any busy medical clinic. Patients are checking in and out at the reception desk, sharing their latest improvements with each other and squealing with excitement. Locals pour in from surrounding neighborhoods. Dr. Shroff treats many of the children for free—some with physical challenges, others with autism and neurological issues. The only patients who are living at the hospital during their treatments are foreigners, like me, who have traveled from other countries—Dubai, Australia, England, New Zealand, and America. Although I did hear that a patient from Florida flew here in his own jet and is staying at the decadent five-star Taj Palace Hotel.

Nutech Mediworld in Green Park is Dr. Shroff's second hospital and opened only this year. Dr. Shroff began her career as an infertility specialist at her original location, in Gautam Nagar, another area of South Delhi that is about ten minutes away. But when she developed her stem cell technology and started treating local patients, word spread and demand grew. To accommodate the onslaught of new international patients, she opened this second hospital, in a newer, more desirable building and location.

I am one of the most able-bodied people at this hospital. The majority of patients have spinal cord injuries and are confined to wheelchairs. I almost feel guilty that I can walk with no assistance, albeit some rocky maneuvering.

Before I can process too much of what I'm seeing, I spot the infamous Dr. Shroff. She is strolling our way in flowing, gauzy clothes, beaming with serenity, in no rush to reach our stuck-together family. She's a mix of saint and rock star—Mother Teresa and Mick Jagger rolled into one. She spells BOSS. Dr. Shroff's very presence demands attention, which she seems completely unaware of. She's turning from side to side, observing peripherally. Her smooth black bob-cut hair is bouncing as she glides in pointed-toe shoes adorned with multicolored beads and sequins. She looks like she's walking down a runway. I've been waiting to meet her for so many months, but suddenly I can't adjust to the reality of it before she reaches us. She is one of the most controversial doctors in the world: to some, a miracle worker, and to others, a peddler of snake oil. She is the last doctor on earth who I believe can help me.

With each new possible treatment or doctor, I've wrestled not only with conflicting opinions but also with my inner voice. I am scared to use my intuition, because I usually can't hear it telling me anything at all, and when I have, it's often been wrong; but I'm equally scared to make random guesses. Choosing to travel here could easily turn out to be my worst decision ever. There are too many reasons to count as to why this might end up being true. But I'll start with this: I am the first Lyme disease patient ever to be treated at this clinic. When I told my Lyme disease specialist at home that I was going to do this, he bit his lip and said, totally straight-faced, "I hope it doesn't kill you."

Doctors in America who specialize in Lyme disease couldn't cure me, and here I am hoping a doctor who has never treated someone with this disease can. I feel the failure of this plan drop in my stomach and smash into pieces.

"Hello," Dr. Shroff says quickly, approaching with a smile. "Please come." Many people here, including some of the hospital staff, don't speak English. Dr. Shroff's is near perfect. She motions down the hall toward her office, and we all follow. We take our seats; I immediately sink deep into the chair cushion and feel it cradle me. Sitting down with Dr. Shroff is only a moment in time, but it weighs a million pounds. If I have led myself to the wrong place, a dangerous place, then there is really nothing left I can trust anymore. This time is different than all that has come before with doctors and treatments galore. There is more at stake—hope, finances, and, dare I say, my ego. I have agreed to blog about my trip on a health-care website that I've occasionally written for. This will make any potential win—or fail—a public spectacle. The pressure of it all suddenly feels insurmountable.

Dad is slightly reclined in his chair. Against his stomach, he is holding a Hindi newspaper that he can't read. He has an insatiable curiosity. He loves people. He loves life. He is epically jolly. Except for when he's not.

When I was ten years old, my mom's dad—my poppy—was dying, and my parents said: "We are going to the hospital to say good-bye now." We piled into our dark blue oversize van with two rotating captain's chair seats, which my siblings and I fought over incessantly, and we set off for the good-bye. The navy velvet interior of the van made it feel like the funeral had already started, and I think it had, because Poppy was gone in a matter of days after that.

It was not too long after Poppy died that my dad got sick. Or maybe depressed. No one ever really figured it out. He was so fatigued that he slept for days. He began to have episodes where he cried loudly and inconsolably out of the blue. None of it made any sense. He would be perfectly fine, the best dad in the world, telling his jokes, being my pillar of comfort—and then in a flash, his eyes would glaze over and he'd have to go to bed. Sometimes after only a few hours, and sometimes after long, sad weeks, he would spontaneously return to pure joy—a buoy in hopeless, rough seas—and he was back.

The episodes remain a mystery with no cause for their baffling arrivals or unpredictable departures. Over the years, doctors tested every possible diagnosis, checking them off the list one by one: bipolar disorder, depression, PTSD, chronic fatigue. All the doctors agreed to disagree. There were many theories, but no one could give us a definitive answer. Our family does the best we can to bounce with the ups and downs. But here, seeing the light in his face, his eagerness for life emanating from his entire being, I still find myself wondering, as if it's brand new, how it's even possible for someone so high on life to hit extremes so low. I've learned to go with what's here today, though, and today he is good. Mom is sitting beside him, looking his way excitedly, and waiting for Dr. Shroff to kick off our meeting—the best sport ever.

"Welcome," Dr. Shroff starts, through her friendly, fluorescent-pink-lipsticked grin. She is in her late forties, beautiful in a striking way, with giant brown sparkly eyes. After a long, silent smile, she gets straight to business.

Dr. Shroff is a bundle of contradictions, both everything and nothing of what I expected. She is sweet and kind, but blunt and precise with her words.

"Everything we do must be documented," she says, thumbing through my medical records.

In one of my many e-mail exchanges with Dr. Shroff, she explained that the Indian Health Council only allows her to treat patients labeled incurable or terminally ill. Her patent-pending stem cell treatment has not gone through the testing and government approval that would make it widely available. Because of this, it carries great risks. For now, only those who cannot be cured by any other means are accepted. Lyme disease, at this stage, and in my case, is considered incurable. I am a person who the government says can take the risk. They agree—I am screwed, and therefore, government-approved stem cell worthy.

Stem cells are a special type of undifferentiated cells, meaning they have the potential to develop into many different types of cells in the body—to make muscles, organs, and more. They could be considered the "wild card" of cells, as they are so versatile. They continue to divide inside the body, providing an internal repair system for damaged cells. I need these cells and am relieved to be incurable, because that's the only way I can get them. A ridiculous oxymoron.

"There is no Lyme disease in India," Dr. Shroff says, "but I did have one Indian patient who had it. He probably contracted it in the US." I wonder how this patient with Lyme is doing, if he or she is even still alive, but I decide against digging further. "Let's just see what happens with you," she says nonchalantly. My chest tenses at the reminder that Dr. Shroff might not know what she is doing with me. Mom, Dad, and I made an agreement before we left home, that if something didn't feel right when we got here, we'd leave. I wonder if either of them is going to stand up now.

"We will get our own baseline and then compare later," she says. Dad chimes in and jokes, "You need proof for your critics, right?" She smirks and looks up. "Oh, the world is my critic." Based on my research about her, this is accurate. The scientific community around the globe is scrutinizing her.

"Nobody believes what I'm doing is real," Dr. Shroff says, leading the conversation toward the specifics of her unique technique. "Just because they don't know *how* I am doing this, they think it cannot be done."

First, Dr. Shroff explains that her cells are pure human embryonic stem cells, meaning that there are no animal products used in her process. This is an anomaly in the world of stem cell technology. "None of my patients have shown any adverse side effects because it is pure," Dr. Shroff says. I both like this and am suspicious of it as well, because based on my past experience, the promise of no side effects sounds impossible. Next, Dr. Shroff claims she is creating her stem cell lines in a way that no other scientist has been able to replicate: she is using and reusing a single embryo to create enough stem cell lines to treat hundreds of patients. "I only use one embryo for all," she states with confidence, her pointer finger proudly displayed. Her technology involves using an original donated embryo over and over in its current phase, never destroying anything at all. "This embryo was given by a generous woman, who after conceiving her two children via IVF wanted to help others," she adds.

Embryonic stem cells are a very controversial subject on their own, but add an Indian female doctor who says she's doing something in a way that other scientists can't figure out, and you have a firestorm.

When the average person thinks about embryonic stem cells, their brain may conjure up scary images of aborted fetuses, political protests, and religious arguments. But this is nowhere close to the reality of it. An embryo at the early stage during which stem cells are extracted is scientifically known as a blastocyst, which is only a few cells.

The blastocyst is approximately 0.1 to 0.2 millimeters, the size of the period at the end of this sentence. Yes, that sentence you just read.

Unused embryos are discarded every day in fertility clinics. Britain's Human Fertilisation and Embryology Authority (HFEA), which has recorded IVF processes since 1991, estimates 1.7 million embryos have been discarded thus far.

Scientists around the world warn that the biggest risk associated with embryonic stem cells is teratomas—noncancerous tumors made up of tissues such as hair, teeth, muscle, and bone. I have to ask her about this, even though I've read online that she says this is not a risk with her patients. Still, I do it fearfully, petrified of her response. If I don't like the answer (I mean, *teeth and bones*?!), will I leave? I am trying to be responsible by being smart and assertive, but the truth is that I don't think anything she would say could change my mind right now. Okay, except maybe *teeth and bones*!

"I've read that because of how you process the stem cells, there is no risk of teratoma tumors, right?" I squish my face in hope. "I keep reading warnings about them and I just want to—"

She jumps in quickly. "This risk is not so with my cells. These scientists are using mice for testing. They cannot know what happens in a human. How can they?" I don't know and don't answer. "By mixing embryonic stem cells with the genetics of a mouse, they are doing something unnatural. This is setting off the wrong reaction. The same would happen if we put mouse cells into our human bodies." She reminds us that her stem cells are a purely human product, which is being transplanted into humans—and therefore, the body accepts it. Our conversation about mice and experiments feels ironic, because I seem like the real lab rat right now. But her explanation makes logical sense, so I let it go.

Next we talk about exactly how the stem cells might help me. The idea behind the treatment is two-part. By strengthening my immune system, Dr. Shroff predicts my body will finally be able to fight some of whatever infection I still have left, on its own. Up until now, my immune system has been so degenerated that it's all been up to the various medications. The new stem cells will also help to reverse the years of damage done to my body from the Lyme disease: damaged nerves, tissues, organs, and more. But this is all theoretical, based on what we know stem cells *can* do. We don't know what they actually *will* do. I am reminded of the words from my Lyme specialist now: "I hope it doesn't kill you." Dr. Shroff explains that the stem cells will keep developing, and working, for up to five years. So she says that even if I don't see immediate improvement, there is still hope to look forward to. I am not sure how to interpret this—should I feel freed of some pressure to show immediate improvement, or worried that she is relieving herself of some responsibility? "There are no guarantees," she says, and then moves on swiftly.

"Okay then. You will need tests so I get my own baseline. I do understand you've been tested thoroughly at home, but we'll do them again. We'll get those scheduled in the next days." Dr. Shroff shows me a list of about fifteen tests, among them a spinal MRI, various blood tests including some special immune-function ones my doctor at home does, a "Doppler" (a.k.a. ultrasound) of my legs, a mammogram, and the list goes on. For the $30,000 I wired to her for the treatment—which, by the way, was the most frightening banking experience of my life—I get room and board at the hospital and all treatment included. Tests are extra. But I am comforted to find out that all the tests will amount to just $1,000. At home, an MRI alone is $2,500. I cannot believe the difference. While these costs may seem astronomical to those who aren't stuck in the loop of the medical system, to me, they are a bargain. Even the $30,000 is a deal if it works. Each year, my family has struggled to pay the gargantuan price tag associated with Lyme disease treatment, which is often not covered by health insurance. If this is the last year we have to do that, I've just hit the jackpot.

"Let's go," she says. It's time for the next part of the orientation tour! "We will go to physio."

I am still processing all the information as we take the stuffy elevator down to the basement physical therapy room, called physio here. It's a large room, dripping with cheery colors that tend more toward neon than primary—fluorescent yellows and brilliant blues that could blind the disease right out of you. Hindi rap music sets the mood, reverberating through the floor, up through my feet. There are other patients well into their sessions. Nyla, a young Indian woman who is rail-thin and frail, is getting this therapy for a heart condition. She doesn't speak English, but smiles when we're introduced. Brian, a twentysomething guy from Australia, is trying to regain use of his legs after a motorcycle accident. He dances with his shoulders and chest, the rest of his body paralyzed and lifeless. An older man, Bob, is using calipers (the Indian version of leg braces) to stand for the first time since he was paralyzed, admiring his accomplishment in the full-length mirror.

The room is busy—the patients and staff are laughing, some are sweating, and I am tired just looking around. I haven't exercised in longer than I can remember. In fact, the last time I did physical therapy, I was too sick and weak to do anything on land so I was prescribed aquatic therapy—a.k.a. "pool school." Five days a week at the physical therapy center, I climbed into the pool, four feet deep and a delightful ninety-four degrees. It was pure relief to my aching body. My pool mates were sick and mostly over seventy, except for the teacher, whose job it was to make sure we didn't drown, and to direct us toward the proper way of doing leg lifts and shoulder shrugs. There was always someone in class cheating, which seemed a total waste of cheating to me. It was pretty much a chlorine melting pot of complainers: Gretchen, who hated her grown kids and had two bad knees; Tom, who hated Gretchen; and Sally, who drove fifteen minutes to get there and spent the first fifteen minutes complaining about her ride. I was not a fan of the group format. In fact, I had only one comrade: eighty-two-year-old Art, who towered over me (although that doesn't take much) and was built like a linebacker. The first time I met Art, I kind of fell in love with him—which is awkward, because when you meet people at pool school, you're both half-naked. He called our pool school buddies "a bunch of hoodlums," and I agreed. He reminded me of Poppy, never taking himself or anything too seriously. Art sported a huge scar from his belly button ascending into the middle of his chest. "I survived some crazy shit," he told me that first day in the locker area. "Almost died," he said, as if the issue were no bigger deal than the weightless leg lifts we'd just done. "Then, after open heart surgery, they finally sewed me up, and I had the most powerful sneeze ever. Those damn stitches unripped like a zipper right up me." Art laughed deeply, like he was hearing about his own ridiculous bad luck for the first time. Every day when we said good-bye, he'd tell me, "Wear your sweatshirt, kid. Things can change pretty fast out there when you least expect it. Life can be funny that way." Still some of my favorite advice.

Here in this physio room, I am happy to see the crowd is mostly *under* seventy and no one is wearing a bathing suit. I heave a deep sigh of relief when I realize each patient has his or her very own physical therapist, and there are no group lessons! I am winning already.

Dr. Shroff introduces me to Chavi, who will be my physical therapist for the entire eight weeks I'm here. She is almost exactly my height, with long, jet-black hair, perfectly aligned teeth, and a round friendly face. She shakes my hand lightly and giggles.

"Let's see what you can do. Fine?" Chavi directs, patting the bed next to her for me to lie down on. Every time she moves my legs even an inch, she smiles at me and says, "Fine?" People here use the word "fine" in abundance, just as we say "okay?" I've already caught on. They understand that "fine" means *move on*, *all done*, *it's all good*, and a host of other things. It gets the point across for almost anything.

The truth is that I haven't been fine with anything for a long, long time—my life, my body, or especially my legs. These legs that are supposed to keep me up have only dragged me down. Their message: *You have no hope to stand on*. It was early 2006, only two years earlier, that I wanted nothing to do with them ever again—my own legs, my mortal enemies.

My parents' back bedroom, which used to belong to my older sister, had become an infirmary where my failing body and the fiercest part of my spirit were housed. Jay and I had moved in when we realized we needed help—financially and emotionally—to be able to survive this new life with my illness.

"You have to do it . . . pleeeease," I begged, lying in the bedroom one evening. That day felt so long it seemed that three days had been crammed into one.

My eyes barely open, thrashing my helpless legs around hard in the tangled sheets, I wailed. I tried my plea again, with added determination. "Cut them off!"

Sitting on the edge of the bed, Jay stared somewhere beyond me. His emotional pain matched my physical pain, but he didn't respond to me at all.

"Do it for me . . . you have to," I sobbed. "I need you to do this."

I don't know what kind of woman begs a man to cut off her legs. I only know that I would have never imagined myself to be her. But somehow, in my desperate and daring state, removing my limbs seemed the only solution to end my unthinkable, atrocious, dire pain.

Searing, slashing, stabbing, burning, without warning.

It felt like a villain from a horror movie was hammering nails into my legs, deeper and harder to test my ability for survival. This agony was caused by a rare form of neuropathy, which is, essentially, damage to the nerves. For months nonstop, I'd been taking eighteen narcotic painkillers in each twenty-four-hour period, yet they hardly touched this pain. The outer sheath of my nerves was unraveling, and doctors couldn't figure out how to stop it. Life was a brand-new kind of impossible.

Removing my legs, I was convinced, was the only logical option. The only option left, really, to save me from the torture. I was fully aware of what I was asking—the seriousness of it, the grossness of it, the sadness of it—but that didn't slow me down. This dramatic episode was not new in our bedroom, but it is the worst I will ever remember.

This man had helped me take baths and restitched my leg with his bare hands after a botched muscle biopsy, and was just as terrified as I was about my future. If anyone would get it, it would be him. He would see my logic, I believed, because I am a logical person and because there was no other choice. He would find solace in the fact that I didn't want to end my life. I didn't want to die. I was *only* asking for my legs to be removed. The only thing I needed was for him to do it.

Turning to me, he finally met my eyes and seemed to absorb what I was asking. He broke. A tear rolled out of each eye. The wetness of his face unexpectedly woke me into reality. I put a halt to my pleading, spontaneously and involuntarily, as if a wall with the word *STOP* moved quickly to meet me. *Stop. Just stop. Stop it*, I heard in my head.

"No," Jay said, the tears coming faster and faster. He would not cut off my legs.

What I realized in that moment is that there are many things we do for love. We will forgo our lives to help another person go on. We will sit by and watch the demise of another's lovely body, anchoring ourselves into happier memories just to survive it. We will tell ourselves that one day, soon, everything will be fine!, even though we know it probably won't be. But there are many things, because of love, we just cannot do. His tears hit my calves, and for only a few seconds, I was grateful I still had them.

In a lifetime of moments, we accrue many ugly ones. It is these moments—the ones that immediately jump to mind in a mental review of our lives—that carry the most shame with them. This is not because we necessarily behaved badly or wrongly, but because we allowed our scariest human insides to show on the outside. The unfiltered-ness of ourselves seeps out. Jay was the person who witnessed the deepest and most desperate parts of me at the exact same time that I discovered them for myself. When there is another person to witness the ugly, you are forced to stare yourself down, right where you are—out in the wide-open, bare to those beside you. Those moments become a crack in your heart, a nail in your coffin, a smudge in your otherwise shiny past. Begging Jay to cut off my legs with his own bare hands will always be my most glaring queen of ugly in a timeline of many. His witness to my insides still shakes me as I watch Chavi twist my legs and measure my nonexistent muscles. Jay and I hardly speak anymore, but I still feel that day strung between us.

Here in physio, I am forced to face the legs I have felt so resentful toward and detached from. As I watch Chavi bending and stretching my deconditioned body, I suddenly understand. When you really love something, you have to be Jay. You have to say no to removing the parts that are ugly. You have to say yes: yes to acceptance, yes to the ugly, and yes to love.

When Dr. Shroff asks if I can get off the physio bed and stand, I do it. I own each foot as it hits the floor. These are my first moments of forgiving my legs, in all of their hideous glory. After years of wishing them away, I take them as mine, just as Jay did.

I try to walk in a line with my eyes open, then with my eyes closed. I fail horribly—veering to the left like a drunken sailor, without the hat or the fun of a drink. The left side of my body is full of bruises from the constant deviations when I can't quite control my stride and accidentally bump into parked cars, unsuspecting furniture, or walls. This impaired balance is caused by decreased blood flow and oxygen to my brain and is a common neurologic symptom in patients with late-stage Lyme disease. Over time, it can cause irreversible brain damage. The symptoms include memory loss, sleep disturbance, fatigue, depression, and, as is on show here, wonky balance. I lean on a chair to catch myself and cock my head with a smile at Dr. Shroff. I'm taking this balancing defeat more lightly than usual because I'm hoping it will be fixed soon.

Dr. Shroff isn't shocked, bothered, or intimidated by any of what I cannot do. She doesn't compare me to the other patients, tell me I'm the worst case of this-or-that that she's ever seen, say that this will be difficult to fix, or anything I've heard from doctors in the past. She also doesn't compare me to my old self, because she has no idea that I was once a person who would hike every weekend, with stamina that my now twenty-pounds-underweight body could never endure. She makes no comments and shows no emotional reactions as she watches me fail, exercise after exercise. Instead of being self-conscious, I find comfort in her blasé observation of me and my dysfunction.

The first days in physio will begin the rebuilding of many things: my muscles and my strength, but mostly the slow awakening of my own self-acceptance—the subtle sense that something inside of me is already more okay than I ever thought.

"I'll see you here tomorrow, fine?" Dr. Shroff says, jotting down a quick note. "Fine!" I confirm. She smiles at Chavi and me and walks away.

•   •   •

"ARE YOU READY?!" Dr. Ashish asks with almost a song, holding the golden needle with a dose of stem cells in his sturdy hand. I am surprised at how fast things are moving here. India does not allow for gentle acclimations. Everything is rushing toward me. I just got here *yesterday*, am admittedly still slightly worried about tumors, and am jet-lagged beyond recognition. I am not by any means ready. But I agree because it is both too early and too late in this game to not be ready.

Dr. Ashish is buoyant. His glasses magnify the excitement in his eyes as he gives the needle the attention it deserves, holding it to the light and beaming at it proudly. It is already time for my very first dose of stem cells and apparently Dr. Ashish is The Man when it comes to this department. Following him is a gang of sisters to assist. I'm excited! I'm hopeful! I am nervous this could kill me!

My parents are sitting in the corner of my hospital room, Dad aiming his camera at the significant moment that is about to occur. He bought a new camera for this trip and has three different manuals and six lenses laid out in front of him. He tells me that he is using both the constant shooting mode and the filming mode. He has prepared to capture this momentous occasion in every way possible. Dr. Ashish is impressed. "Isn't that clever!" he says. My mom is overwhelmed with emotion, lips pressed tight, as if she's about to witness a birth. She could care less about the camera's advanced functions.

"We are doing a test dose only to make sure there is no reaction," Dr. Ashish says. He delivers this news with a look of concern, brow furrowed, and I feel myself worry. "We are looking for a rash at the injection site," he finishes. A laugh breaks through my lips. After all I've been through, a rash would be the least of my problems.

There are three parts to making sure these cells have the best chance, Dr. Ashish explains. "They will be influenced in part by physiotherapy, part will be your mind and spirit, and the rest will be how your body reacts on its own: fate." He is counting the parts off on his fingers as he speaks. "Your attitude, nurturing, and positivity must be there! You have an approximate twenty percent influence," Dr. Ashish specifies deliberately with great intent.

"These cells are immature and need to be trained to function properly. Embryonic, if you will!" Dr. Ashish waits for us to laugh at his joke. I feel Dad zoom in on my face with his super-lens.

"I understand," I promise. I don't take it on, but I do take it in. "These cells will have a good home."

I feel a twinge of emotion in my chest and a sting in my throat like I might cry. I hold back. I can't wait until he does the injection and they are mine to keep.

Slowly, Dr. Ashish wipes the inside of my right bicep to prepare for the injection. "This will be a prick," he explains. I feel my dad zooming in from behind the camera. Dr. Ashish finally, slowly injects a syringe full of clear liquid into my arm. "Fine?!" he asks. I feel nothing and am slightly let down by how fast the moment passes. There is no rainbow that appears over me, no Oompa-Loompas who come out singing, and no confetti that falls from the sky.

"Fine!" I tell him.

"Now, we cannot know exactly where these cells will go!" he says. "They will find homes in the tissues where they are needed to begin regeneration. Very intelligent."

I hope this isn't like when you lose weight and try so hard to direct any fat-burning to your hips, thighs, and stomach—but your body decides to target it all to your boobs. I send a silent message to the stem cells in case they are listening: *Ignore my boobs. Please go directly to my legs.*

These cells will be administered daily, first by injection like now and then by IV so they can give me larger doses.

As he leaves, Dr. Ashish gives me a list of directions: eat more than normal, don't do anything that might harm the stem cells, and get plenty of rest. I am already nervous that I'll tilt the cells the wrong way or something and screw this up. This treatment has to work.

I lie perfectly still and try to settle into the moment, listening to my parents' comforting chatter in the background, but the rambunctious street below is roaring. I picture it celebrating with me. India is calling me out of my room, out to meet my brand-new city.

Two extra Percocet and twenty minutes later, the three of us are jammed in the bench seat of a tuk-tuk for a wind-blown, loud, wild ride to a local market. When I was growing up, we would set off on family drives with no predetermined destination, sometimes getting lost in exploration. As we kids started to get nervous about being in the middle of nowhere, my dad would lighten the mood and say, "It's just a zoomy ride!" But this ride has been a zoomy one from the start and Dad is holding on for dear life. I guess a zoomy ride is not as fun when you're not behind the wheel. This open-air cart feels like it could tip every time it turns a corner, and none of us know our way. The sky is black, full of soot, as if a chemical storm is brewing, and the only discernible marker of where we are is the sun behind it, which is a vivid blood orange.

The market has the look and feel of a traditional rural

village bazaar. There are rows of colorful stalls squished right up next to each other, arranged around a dusty courtyard. Children hustle beaded necklaces that hang from their arms, men sell roasted sweet potatoes, and women chat. Every woman in India is draped in gorgeous fabrics and jewelry, with perfectly done hair. I am wearing jeans, a hoodie, and a backpack. None of me is sparkling, shining, or shimmering.

The market allots stalls to craftspeople from different parts of India on a rotational basis of fifteen days, so there is always something new for visitors to marvel at. Inside, people are busily shopping for handicrafts and the vendors call us into their stalls as we meander, offering us a variety of things they are convinced we need.

"Hello, ma'am! You must see my stepstool!" one woman hollers, stepping up and down from it repeatedly as if it's the perfect makeshift exercise stair-stepper. Another lady, holding a giant men's T-shirt, calls to me: "Ma'am, this shirt has been waiting for you! Take a look, ma'am." I am overpowered and underprepared for this experience. There are people coming at me from every direction. When I turn around to find my parents, I see my dad playing a flute in front of the next booth—a crowd of Indian families with children encircling him, jumping and cheering. This geeky and totally charming American is the most popular attraction at the market.

I kindly say "No thank you" to several different food vendors for what feels like at least four hundred times. The authentic food from various regions in India smells . . . interesting, or spicy, or something that I can't really identify. A sweet older lady urges me to try the *momos* from the hilly state of Sikkim, India. *Momos* are a South Asian dumpling, often filled with onion, garlic, and coriander. I'm tempted, but I've been warned against eating the street food here, even though I probably have enough antibiotics in my system from treating Lyme to kill any foreign invader—well, except the Lyme, which seems to survive everything and anything.

As I roam through this market, it is all brand-new. Here, I am an outsider with the unanticipated relief of already not fitting in. I don't even have a chance of doing so. No one expects anything from me, which makes me less aware of how bad I feel—the shakiness in my legs from fatigue, pain contracting my entire body, and my heart beating at what feels like twice the normal rate.

In the days after I first got sick, and when I was trying hardest to hang on, to both my legs and my sanity, my friend Mandy would drag me out to the bar to watch football with our group of friends. I sat at the table and chased my painkillers with beer. I tried to be the girl I once was and the girlfriend Jay had signed up for.

It was usually not long before I ran out of patience for

the struggle it was to survive outside the house, but I continued to do it. I am still not entirely sure why. Either I recognized that practicing life, even when you feel shut out from it, is an essential part of not completely losing your footing in it—or I was determined, despite my lack of ability, to still be who I wished I were. This practice felt both simultaneously healthy and also like an enormous self-imposed extra pressure.

In those days, it was difficult to identify how I was really feeling because as I'd always been, I was most concerned with how everyone else was feeling. My worries about how my being sick was affecting my family and my friends were pulling me apart inside. I was, in many respects, desperate to stay in the game and show the people around me that I was fine. But what I really wanted to do, and very much needed to do, was curl up in my bed, guilt-free. I spent my life oscillating between two realities: a force who was drawn to taking care of and pleasing others; and a person who was constantly making failed efforts to say a hard-and-fast no to things that I kept saying yes to: social obligations instead of the copious amounts of alone time I craved, helping people when I was drained myself, and generally forcing myself to be whoever I thought the world needed me to be. Either I was never aware of what I needed or I was willing to forgo it at all costs. Probably both. At that time, though, the pressure of all I was trying to keep up with was not only causing inner turmoil but also crushing me further into physical decline.

Here, without my own or others' attachments to who I was, am, or should be, I can be anything. Here, I am nobody. I am new again—free, just as I am.

After a loop through every aisle of the market, I circle back to a booth selling hundreds of elephant figurines—made from wood, clay, and metal, painted in bright rainbow colors. Elephant statues of all sizes are a common sight in India, strong symbols of wisdom, good fortune, new beginnings, and success. They are especially prominent in the form of the Hindu elephant-headed god Ganesh (or Ganesha), who is said to be the remover of obstacles. I see them prominently displayed in the hospital lobby, in the windows of shops and restaurants, on the steps of temples, and sometimes on the side of the street where they don't belong to anybody at all. I feel like I need my own little elephant—a declaration of overcoming obstacles. I spot one just a few inches high, staring right at me. She is firmly planted on all four feet, her body painted in blue, orange, pink, and green, with her trunk shooting up toward the sky in unwavering confidence. I buy it with the help of two friendly Indian women who teach me how to bargain; the shopkeeper wraps it in tissue paper, and I walk off proudly with my very first Indian souvenir.

As we exit through the gates of the market, a woman

and her baby follow us, asking for money. They trail for blocks and blocks. I try to continue walking, ignoring the constant calls and tugs at my heart, but they see through me and call directly to the natural-born saver and obsessive-compulsive rescuer at my core. I empty all the coins from my pocket, which feels like not nearly enough, and without notice five more beggars appear out of nowhere, telling us different stories at once: they need food for their baby, mother, brother, dog, or goat. They must have a secret code for *Hey, come quick because we've got a sucker on our hands.*

My first full week here is much like this first outing. Everything is moving lightning fast and none of it is familiar, but I am okay anyway. I am completely calm, present, and surprised at this comfort I feel in my new world, and even in my own skin. Each day, I get my morning stem cells either by shot or via IV. Chills flood through my lower body like sheets of rain. I imagine the cells fixing every inch of me. After my stem cell dose, I go to physio, where Chavi cheerleads me through even the smallest accomplishments. I tire after five leg lifts, but she is still proud. Some afternoons I rest, and some days Mom, Dad, and I sneak back out onto the streets when I feel well enough. The sisters love to see what treasures we come back with so they can determine whether we got a fair bargain. I lay the items out on my bed and they examine each carefully, either with pleasure or great disappointment. I now have a new dress ("Smart!" they say, which means *fancy* here), dangly earrings (thumbs down, as they tell me cheap jewelry here is full of lead), and a small terra-cotta Ganesha figurine (they approve).

Having made it to this point, I do not have any desire to change my priorities or wishes about the future. I still don't want anything grand or spectacular for my life. I long to wake up in the morning and get out of bed without aching in the deepest parts of my bones. I want to have enough energy to do more than one errand at a time. I want to roll over without excruciating pain following my every move. I want to travel without worrying about taking an entire suitcase for medicine, and having to arrange wheelchair service. Mostly, I want to feel strong enough to play with my two-year-old nephew, Zach—who has Lauren's shiny brown eyes, her husband Craig's patience, and a heart full of joy. He is the first baby in our family and the little light of my life. I want to be fully engaged in life with him.

I often look around and wonder what it would be like to feel healthy again. I never realized, until I was without it, that health is not a state of being or a goal to be attained, but rather a distinct *feeling*. Chronic illness does not delete who you are, it covers up who you are. It lays upon you hundreds of pounds of useless weight, crushing something deep inside. Being sick does not change the person you are—but it does make being that person a whole lot harder. For now, the feeling of health is elusive and something I can only imagine; but it is not something I'll ever give up on finding.

When dusk arrives each night, smoke floods the grayish-pink sky and erases the receding sun. I am hypnotized listening to people chant from the Sikh temple at the end of the street. In my ocean-blue room on the other side of the world from all that I know, I am both wildly chained to my circumstances and also freer than perhaps I've ever been. If I could be doing anything in the world right now, there is nothing I'd choose over this. Absolutely nothing.

I feel full of life in a new sort of way. My emotions seem slightly closer to the surface, a place they do not normally sit, forcing me to acknowledge the bigness, hopefulness of what is happening to me. If I could freeze moments in time, these would be them.

3

A Solid, Unshakable, Pragmatic ROCK

WEEK TWO

I am losing my ever-loving mind. This is code red, full-on freak-outs-ville. To put it nicely, my honeymoon period in India is over.

I am the person who can get through any crisis. I am a tree. I am steel. I am unbreakable. I am a solid, unshakable, pragmatic rock. Except now.

I am falling the fuck apart.

There have been days with no hot water, which stops me not only from showering but also from washing my dishes and my underwear—both of which I have to do *in* the shower. The intermittent Internet access cuts me off from my lifeline to home. Then there is the noise. Ohmyholycow, the *noise*. Even after dark, there is not a second that's quiet. Honking horns. Yelling people. Beeping trucks. Howling dogs. Screaming children. Cars backfiring. Motorcycles skidding out. For someone whose own thoughts are loud and disruptive enough, this external pandemonium has posed quite a challenge. I have always had impeccable hearing. When I was a kid, I could hear the dog-training devices that are supposed to be silent to the human ear. In the past few years, I have become even more noise-sensitive—another symptom of Lyme disease. I register everything at what feels like a billion decibels.

I am also totally unable to find any kind of peace with the food here. The stem cells are kicking my appetite into high gear, and I can't get full or satisfied no matter how hard I try.

The hospital chefs do their best to accommodate the foreign patients by serving "American food," but the spaghetti Bolognese has curry sauce on it, there is corn in everything, and I often cannot identify what the spongy carb on my plate is. When meals are served in my room each day, I pick at whatever of it I can stand to eat, even though I am starving. My friends at home often call me Sally—as in *When Harry Met Sally*. Everything I eat is ordered on the side, without this or that, or altered in some way. This is just not a great place to be Sally. I am my own worst food enemy.

Dr. Shroff has kindly offered to have Indian food sent

from her other hospital in Gautam Nagar, where they only care for local patients and only serve authentic food. She promises the chef is fantastic and everyone there is pleased with the meals. I have no doubt about this at all, but the problem is that I'm not a big fan of Indian food. When I decided to come here for treatment, one of my first thoughts was, *Why, oh why can't it be in China?* I *love* Chinese food.

I had never even tried Indian food before I made the decision to come to Delhi. After I booked my flight, my friend Ajay, whose family is from Udaipur in southern Rajasthan, said, "Amy, the first time you eat Indian food *cannot* be in India." Thank goodness for Ajay. He took me out to his favorite local Indian restaurant, where the hammering Hindi music and pungent waves of cardamom fought for space in the air. The dining room was draped in gold-colored curtains and scattered with silky burgundy pillows. The set of shelves behind the hostess desk showed off several framed pictures and figurines depicting Hindu gods and goddesses. Everywhere I looked, there was something to see. Except on the menu. When we sat down at our table, I couldn't find a single dish that could be ordered Sally-style. Ajay did the ordering: *saag aloo*, potatoes and spinach cooked with garlic, ginger, and chili; *butter chicken*, tender pieces of chicken in a rich butter and tomato sauce; and *tandoori seekh kebab*, ground lamb cooked on skewers in a special clay oven. While I did end up kinda liking my meal, I still only ate half the plate. I should have known I'd be in trouble when I hit the real world. I wish now that I had tried harder not only to be okay with Indian food, but to *love* it. I regret not going back every week to try another dish as if I were training for a marathon . . . of Indian spices. By the cash register, there was a small bowl of fragrant colored confetti that people were scooping into their hands with a tiny spoon and putting in their mouths. *Mukhwas* is a type of breath freshener and digestion aide that includes candy-coated fennel seeds, called *saunf* in Hindi. It's like eating perfume, but better. This, I *loved*. But surviving on breath freshener for my entire time here is less than ideal.

In an effort to meet the goal of satiety, I've had to get culinarily creative, making food in the electric kettle in my room: rice, boiled carrots, and soup. Desperation is the mother of invention. I get my vegetables from a man selling them from a wooden cart on a street corner. I clean each of the ingredients with antibacterial wipes before eating or cooking them, just for extra protection against bacteria and food-borne illnesses. I buy the rest of the items I need from a grocery store close by. It looks like a corner store you might see in New York City, but with a seriously Indian twist. Food items are literally piled on top of each other from floor to ceiling—boxes, bags, and cans—in no orderly fashion. When I pick something out, everything around it falls down. I'm clearly not yet skilled enough to navigate the Jenga puzzle of the shelfless markets. Cartons of eggs are piled five feet high and labeled "Keggs." The "Keggs" have a sticker on them that says "nearly organic." My parents and I have gone around and around trying to figure out what the "K" in Keggs stands for (Kreative, maybe?), but we're no closer to solving the mystery than when we started. I eat three or four of them a day anyway.

Even though the doctors reassure me that hunger is a side effect of the stem cell treatments, I wonder if my struggle with it is also a deeper message from my soul. What am I really so hungry for? At this rate, the answer could be . . . everything. I am hungry for the comfort of my own bed, the silence of nature, and socks that aren't permanently stained from the soot on my hospital room floor, for some kind of control over my food, and for my former mental stability.

Living with a rat in my room has not been helping matters either. The first time I heard its nails scurry on the windowsill, it was just after midnight and it was inches from my head. I shot out of bed in terror, deciding what I should do. Call the front desk? Sleep in the bathroom? Instead, I was kept awake in distress and starving, listening to her eat my crackers. I assume only a *she* would be so perpetually insistent.

Instead of reporting this intruder to the hospital staff, I do what I always do when I can't figure something out— try to see if maybe it's some kind of sign from the Universe.

It was while I was visiting my brother, David, in New York City that I had my very first phone meeting with Dr. Shroff—the one that would close the space between me and my wide-open future. "You may come to India as soon as possible," she confirmed after studying my medical records. Her approval felt like the equivalent of a never-ending ladder in a game of Chutes and Ladders. Was I really getting to climb ahead of science and time toward a cutting-edge medical treatment I couldn't get in the US? Just that morning, David had had to help lift me up off the bedroom floor when I couldn't get up on my own.

The following day on my way back to the airport, my cab encountered an ugly construction mess, which detoured us one quick street over. As I looked out through the fogged-up backseat window, my jaw fell in awe. As far as I could see, the entire street was lined with fuchsia flags that danced in the wind and read: *Incredible India!*

That's when I became hyper-cognizant that in the little flashes of life, there are signs everywhere. I've been looking more closely ever since.

The interpretations I find online about rats are actually quite intriguing. First, that a rat has scurried across your path may mean you need to assert yourself in new ways.

Hmm, could be true. Another possible symbolism is "new beginnings." Definitely feels right. Then I find something that has been observed for centuries: the proverbial notion that rats can tell when a ship is sinking and possess a mystical power to anticipate disaster. Seriously, Universe? This is terrifying. Is the rat here to tell me to hurry up and flee this place before it's too late? Or has she made a home here because she's telling me I should stay? Now she is not only my annoying roommate, but a cryptic messenger. It's been a week now and the point of her presence is still not clear. After I finally tell the front desk about my new hairy sign from the Universe, the staff, unbeknownst to me, set a makeshift glue trap. But the only thing it catches is my now-sacrificed furry and jeweled purple slipper. The rodent still runs free, so now we are roommates during the day, but at night I sleep in a safe zone, the hospital room next door. The rat is clearly winning.

But all of that—the lack of hot water, the noise, the food drama, the rat—is only what's going on *outside* of me. The inside of me is also in complete chaos.

I feel like a massive contradiction, parts of me healing and surviving and other parts synchronistically coming undone. At this time in my life, I have not yet learned that this is almost always how we get from one place in our lives to the next: very, very messily.

Despite my goal of getting off all of these medications

I take, I've had to start several new antibiotics to protect my new stem cells from getting infected with Lyme. I feel even more heavy and exhausted than before and am not sure if it's the Lyme getting kicked up, or the new meds dragging me down.

There is a common phenomenon that occurs with Lyme disease treatment called a Herxheimer (herx) reaction. This reaction happens when the Lyme bacteria die off and other toxins are released in the body. During this time, symptoms may flare while the body works hard to eliminate the toxins and recalibrate itself. The process feels terrible, but is seen as a positive indication that the treatment is working. No pain, no gain?

Dr. Ashish has also told me about a concept called retracing. "When you are getting well, you may go backward, often re-experiencing symptoms in the opposite chronological order they first appeared!" he explains. He is fascinated and excited by this process. "The first symptoms to come will be the last to go, but you may endure them each one more time," he says, raising his eyebrows. So now I am constantly confused about whether the "getting worse" is actually happening because I am getting better. Or maybe I'm just getting worse.

In good news, some of my symptoms are clearly improving! My pain has faded ever so slightly, enough that I've been able to decrease my narcotic pain medication by half a pill per day. When your body is constantly pulsating with pain, any improvement is a huge deal. Like, mega-big. I've also been able to cut back my sleeping medication, and as an extra bonus, I haven't had to take my prescription for heart palpitations, which used to be my constant companion. Since I've been sick, I have only ever added medications. Never have I decreased them—except when they were making me worse or not working at all. When I glance over at my nightstand overflowing with bottles of pills, a small part of me is finally able to entertain the idea that a day might come when I don't need them—or at least, not every single one of them. Every morning and evening when I get my stem cell injections, my muscles begin to twitch, responding with what feels like a happy dance. My heart swells and I'm engulfed with thanks. But still, I am cautiously optimistic. Could I really be improving this quickly? The other day, a group of disgruntled patients who don't think they're getting results fast enough were touting a conspiracy theory that we're getting apple juice in our IVs. But if that's true, those are some damn good apples.

I've been continuing my strength and balance training with Chavi. It finally seems my brain is beginning to get along with my body. I know this because my tendency to veer into walls and bump into mothers carrying small children has subsided. For the first time since I can remember, the left hemisphere of my body is flawlessly intact—no bruises, scrapes, or scratches.

Even though good things are happening, when I'm feeling sick all my improvements get buried. When I am already in a vulnerable place and then get scared, everything hopeful and positive I feel about my body's healing ability seems to get erased. I end up triggered into fear and overwhelm, unable to separate what part of my experience is the symptoms of the disease, what part is the reactions from the treatments, and what part is the real me. Is there even a *real me* anymore?

The doctors here are kind, intelligent, and warm, but it is a challenge even for the best Lyme specialists at home to wrangle this disease. And now I am alone in this foreign land, where Lyme disease doesn't even exist, trying to navigate everything by myself.

This time in India has been an unexpected emotional land mine, my feelings magnified as if they are on a dose of steroids large enough to kill a horse. And I am trying desperately to counteract this by doing what I always do—be stronger, and more in control, than my emotions. But I am ready to produce enough tears at any given moment to bathe a large village of children. I alternate between positive self-talk (*It's okay, you've got this*) and a hearty dose of self-beration (*Seriously, what is wrong with you?!*). Neither is working. I am a mascara-sabotaging mess who should really buy stock in Kleenex. I feel as if some deep inner emotional beast, a side of myself that I've never met, has been unleashed, never to be contained again. I need a user's manual to find its purpose, but am left to survive in these swells of unreliable emotion with no direction. I imagine my current state as an EKG graph where the doctor points to the erratic lines and says, "This line should be all within this range, but see how it's going up and down and up and down?" Then he reaches his finger to indicate the parallel lines of the graph. "We want it more over . . . here."

I am experiencing a discomfort I cannot seem to acclimate to or separate from. The most difficult part of this is that I have a legitimate fear of showing people my less-than-perfect self.

This emotional rawness is different from any physical pain I've ever endured. My body has coping mechanisms for the physical torment now. During some of my most excruciating medical tests and procedures, I managed to distract myself: eyeing the popcorn ceiling above the examination table carefully, trying to find a pattern; cooking imaginary meals in my head; or paying acute attention to each and every noise coming from the hallway. During a bone marrow biopsy years ago, I listened to the powerful, piercing click as the doctor penetrated my pelvic bone with a long hollow needle to take a sample. Despite the pain, I could still distance myself from it, visualizing the removed piece of me being replaced with the sun.

But me right now? I am losing my breath just from being stuck in my own company.

I am the easygoing one, the never-bothered one, the everything-is-great and totally together one. If ever there is someone in need, overcome with sadness, hurt or broken—I am their girl. I'll drop, stop, and spin to light everyone else up and make them feel better. I can usually even hold myself together at the same time. But what I am just now beginning to recognize is that it sometimes takes every ounce of my effort for me to be this person.

It turns out that I am a closet control freak in serious disguise. Inside my head, I am not always so easygoing. I am constantly making plans, figuring things out, analyzing possibilities, and manipulating scenarios to be in control—because control equals safety for me. And my need for safety and stability has always taken precedence over everything else.

I believe that everyone is a mix of two people, or maybe even more: broken and whole, traumatized and fine, a mess and lovely, and, like me, carefully controlled and a free spirit. While I think some of us are born as sensitive souls, I also believe we go through life and things happen, things that make us crack. These cracks feel giant, lonely, as if we are the only one on earth with them. And when we don't know what to do with those cracks, we do anything and everything to keep them buried. But they only grow.

The first real crack I remember is when my dad got sick. With him being up and down and our whole family living on an unpredictable wave, I turned to the conviction that if I could remain okay, we would all be okay. It was then that my need for safety, stability, and a very steady ship became most important, but also least possible to achieve.

Much of my life was about being perfect, mature, compassionate, and good—the quintessential middle child. I am not only the middle child in age, but also smack-dab in the middle of the spectrum between my siblings' personalities. David is the baby of the family—sure, blunt, and unafraid to speak the harsh truth. He is also colossally sweet and exceptionally creative and intelligent. He was always the smartest person I knew, reading books non-stop, even while walking to his friend's house just a few blocks away. We spent our childhood catching lizards and putting on talent shows for our parents. When I was old enough to babysit, he went with me to help. Lauren is the classic older sister. She rules the roost always, rolls her eyes often, and is the kind of sarcastic that gets you addicted to having conversations with her. We have the same cheeks and mannerisms, and laugh hysterically together until we can't breathe. Lauren is authentically friendly, gets shit done, and plays by the rules. You won't meet a person in the world who doesn't say "She's the best!" when you speak her name.

I always strived to be the perfect one, to make my mom and dad happy and proud. I had an incessant worry that I would disappoint them. This, even though they so freely poured unconditional love my way no matter what I did or said. They always made me feel like their special little girl. Smart. Funny. Uniquely me.

I admitted to no one, even myself, what was really going on in my house with my dad, or within myself. *You've got this*, my body decided without any conscious approval from me. *This ship shall not rock.*

It created an involuntary chain reaction within me where I lived my life in a managed, calculated way to ensure my success. I kept the cracks sealed. I started to unconsciously hold my breath. I stuffed all my feelings deep down in my body and I tried to move along with life so nobody would notice. I had anxiety about everything—that my parents would forget to pick me up from school, that our house would get robbed, that we'd get in a car crash—believing, I think, that if I worried enough, I'd catch things before they went wrong.

But there was also another side of me that coexisted, covering up those cracks. And this part of me was just as real as the other. This is the part of me that I almost always am, especially to the outside world, until now, when I'm unraveling at the seams in Delhi.

I was a fun and funny kid and made my parents laugh.

I danced around to sixties music and never looked up to see who was watching. I wanted to become a veterinarian, and then be a housewife, and then decided on medical school, all by the age of eight. I had lots of friends and chased the ice cream truck with neighborhood kids. I was confident with adults, somewhat cool at school depending on whom you ask, and cheerful. I was brave, artistic, and self-assured. I genuinely loved helping people. The only requirements I had for perfection were in my own head.

I grew up and became much the same adult, splitting myself in two. I was about to turn twenty-one when I met Jay, who was older than me by seven years, the same age as Lauren. He had spiky dark hair, a pierced tongue, and a huge upper-back tattoo that announced his last name in ALL CAPITAL LETTERS.

Jay was bold. He was edgy. His feelings were big and he wore them on the outside. He drove his convertible too fast and drank his beers even faster. But for every cool, bad-boy character trait Jay had, there was an intelligent and sensitive one. He painted my toenails and watched B movies on the Hallmark channel with me all weekend. We contemplated deep existential questions: the meaning of life and the concept of karma. His grandma had taught him how to cook, and in turn, he taught me. He also made the best Bloody Mary you've ever had with just the right amount of kick and double the celery, no olives, just the way I like them.

Jay didn't care what anyone thought about him or what he was doing with his life. He was the opposite of everything I want to run from in myself, because Jay was not worried about being safe and perfect. Jay was just Jay. He was the opposite *of* me, which made him a magnet *for* me.

He showed me that life is meant to be fun, from our very first date on a weeknight when we didn't keep track of our beer tab, the number of chicken wing orders, or the clock. We kissed like we were the only two people at the pub. He said no to friends and family without guilt, left work at exactly five o'clock, and treated every day like Friday. Life was a party boat! I jumped on board like it could not capsize.

I decided I would be free, like Jay. I would not worry, like him. I would not care, like him. I would even occasionally forget that my dad, who was now sometimes suicidal from the depression and fatigue, might or might not be alive at any given moment.

I was never without a drink in my hand after work and on the weekends—champagne, Malibu rum, or both. At Jay's encouragement, I stopped flat-ironing my hair, let it curl wildly, and bleached it blond. I traded in my clear gloss for dark crimson lipstick. I wore tighter and trendier clothes. This new life worked. I had never felt so free. But the catch was that I had to keep it up. And the problem that I couldn't see at the time was that this wasn't *me*. The free girl inside, she was all me. But what I had to do to get her out was not.

It was the summer of 2005, five years after Jay and I started dating, when my life busted open at every possible seam.

Mexico and margaritas: the perfect combination. I was sitting in the bubbling hot tub at our gorgeous hotel in Puerto Vallarta, a frosty pink salt-rimmed drink in my hand, watching the sun kiss the beach and sweep the sky. The soft breeze was carrying all my worries away as I swirled my legs around in the water, admiring my cotton-candy-pink nail polish, which matched exactly how I felt. Jay was by my side sipping his own drink, brimming with genuine contentment. Latin music hummed at just the right volume.

This is usually the time in the story when the narrator says, *I never saw it coming.* I think, though, I actually did see things coming, but was a well-trained expert at ignoring them. I have always been very good at not noticing things that I am noticing, if by actually noticing them, my life might get too hard.

It was there in that Jacuzzi in Mexico that my body was about to hijack my life; I'm sure, because I never would have done it on my own.

I was suddenly startled by stabbing pains, from my knees down to my petite feet. "I can't move!" I screamed to Jay, becoming quickly frozen in temporary paralysis. Heat rushed up through my head, making me dizzy, my entire being burning with pure, raging panic. My mind couldn't keep up with what I was feeling—fear, pain, confusion. And in the two minutes we were nervously discussing what could be going on (dehydration! muscle cramps! too much tequila!), the overwhelming pain began to pass. I lifted myself from the water, never releasing my drink from my fingertips.

I think that all the cracks I'd been avoiding for my whole life showed up in my legs all at once. It was only six months later that I was bedridden and begging Jay to cut my legs off.

Here in India, even my cracks are cracking. Everything is erratic, uncertain, and unsafe—including myself. The unstable, sensitive me that I wanted no one to see is pouring out uncontrollably. I am the opposite of what I've worked hard for my entire existence.

What I wish I'd known at this time in my life is that everyone is perfectly fractured. The cracks that I thought were only inside of me are the same cracks that everyone has. And both the cracks and the repair work are half the point of life itself. There is really nothing to run from, nothing to resist at all. But I don't have a clue about any of that in the moments that I'm bawling in the shower louder than the barking dogs in the alley, staring numbly out my window into a world full of tuk-tuk madness and monkeys, and being sent away from physio because I can't stop crying long enough to complete even a single leg lift.

I hesitantly divulge to Dr. Ashish how I feel and find the slightest sense of relief when he tells me, "It is common to have exaggerated emotions with stem cells!" I almost cry (surprise!) at his confirmation.

But I can feel that this is not just stem cells. Maybe the stem cells have pushed open the floodgates, but there is a deep well of emotion that has been sloshing around for a long, long time. Perhaps it is only some ten thousand miles from home that I am finally willing to let it rise.

"Keep your eye on the prize of health!" Dr. Ashish exclaims through his pearly white grin. He reminds me that I have to be gentle with myself, remain positive, and nourish my cells in every way I can. I've always considered myself a positive thinker, proud of how I tend to see, or maybe force myself to see, the glass half full. But I am not great at being kind and gentle with myself. I am not sure how this happened, or when, but the names I call myself and the things I tell myself are not anything I'd ever say to another person. In fact, I never allow myself any slack, a break, the luxury of changing my mind, or an excuse to fall off the perfection wagon. Even so, Dr. Ashish has a way about him that convinces me being softer is the only way to proceed, so onward I'll try.

In fact, I have already started this mission. I've been reading *The Hidden Messages in Water* by the Japanese scientist Masaru Emoto. I tucked this thin book in my suitcase before I left, as a "maybe I'll finally get to this" token gesture.

In the book, Dr. Emoto collects water from various environments and looks at it under a microscope. He takes pictures to show how the molecules react to heavy metal music, positive words, and more. The results are freaky—negative words create muddied-looking asymmetrical patterns, and loving ones create gorgeous crystal formations that resemble snowflakes. The cells in our body are, in large part, water. That means whatever words and emotions influence water, also influence *me*. This is my first hint of understanding that all the pressure I put on myself to be perfect, for me and for everyone else, has got to change.

After my talk with Dr. Ashish, I commit to reading a little from the book every single day. Instead of entertaining my constant fears, frustrations, and failures, I will focus on what causes magnificent crystals to form: gentleness, love, and compassion. What I learn from this book will turn out to be only one microprint in my slow evolution toward internal transformation. Reading it may not create a dramatic turn in events that carries me along with ease from this point on, but I sense it is doing me some sort of good.

While my relationship with Dr. Ashish is effortless and an absolute joy, my interactions with Dr. Shroff are another story (read: *complicated*).

It feels like she has chosen me as her pet project, continuously giving me unsolicited pep talks and advice about my personal power to heal.

"The stem cells can do their part, but you have the power to heal yourself," she tells me one day when I'm trying not to topple off the steps in physio, struggling with intolerable fatigue, and fighting back tears. Then she adds, "You have much more power than you think."

"Amy, remember, you can't be too nice in life or you'll lose yourself," she preaches to me another day in the hallway when I share that I'm worried about a sick friend back home.

The next day when we meet in the hospital lobby, she starts again. "Are you doing better today? Remember, carrying the problems of the world is not a good trait and results in the breakdown of the body." She cheerfully walks away, leaving me with a citation for bad behavior.

"The stem cells can do their part, but you have the power to heal yourself," Dr. Shroff repeats almost daily now, like a broken record I desperately want to stop. My deepest gratitude for her alternates with my intense resentment toward her for pushing what I so naively label *Eastern philosophical bullshit*. In my delicate mental state,

I make master plans to dodge her passing presence in the hallways in order to avoid a total meltdown. She seems to believe that I have some superhuman healing power, which, if true, I can't find anywhere. *My room looks like a bomb hit it*, I sarcastically think during our conversations. *Maybe my power is under my laundry.* Also, *Why the fuck am I here if I can heal myself?*

I'm immersed in an Eastern culture where it is believed that karma plays a part in everything, the mind is undoubtedly the root of any challenge, and if you want something badly enough, you can have it—or if you don't want something, you can wish it away. Of course I desperately want to wish my illness away. So if I can't, where does that leave me?

I wish I could be one of those totally Zen people who are undisturbed by the world around them. I want to weather these storms gracefully and peacefully . . . maybe meditating or sitting in a yoga pose until they pass. Unfortunately, I am the opposite of this right now. I am shaken to the core and my tethers to sanity are slowly slipping away. It has become apparent to me how the amenities and consistencies of home swaddle me in comfort. I think, if someone were complaining to me about these very things that are tormenting me now, I would say to them, "But you might get to live! How bad can the food be? Wear some headphones for the noise! Crying won't kill you!" And maybe even, in a less than compassionate moment, "GET YOURSELF TOGETHER." This is always how it goes, though. It's like sitting in your air-conditioned house deciding you can totally handle camping in the searing desert heat of California's Death Valley. You understand the idea of no running water, a blazing sun, and little shelter, but you think, *I'll drink cold drinks, I'll wear a hat, I'll be fine.* And then you get there and are trapped in a sweaty, suffocating tent where you can hardly breathe. The point is, shit gets real when it's actually happening.

I'm hanging on to the threads that connect me to home, hoping they'll be enough to hold me together: the Skype calls where I watch Zach eat mac and cheese and practice saying "pasta" from his high chair; the encouraging comments left on my blog posts by loved ones, but also strangers who have stumbled onto it; and e-mails from my friends providing updates on the drama in their lives at home. But as grateful as I am for these things, they hardly anchor me. There is only one reason I have not begged my parents to get back on that plane with me and go home: faith.

It was only a year earlier that I was prompted to seriously contemplate the idea of faith, because I needed desperately to believe that there was some greater agenda to my existence than just my suffering. It was essential for me to find some kind of belief that my mess of a life had any order or meaning at all.

Jay and I had landed in Chicago for yet another extreme but promising treatment option. When it turned out to be a dead end, I was thrown into a state of despondency. While I had managed to maintain a mostly decent mind-set up until then, it became apparent that I would need more if I were to survive with any grace. Or survive at all. The big problem was that I wasn't sure exactly what faith was or how to get it. I had always struggled with the idea of faith: unfettered belief that is not based on any proof. I speak the language of logic and science. I often wondered how people develop the blind trust that faith requires. Where does it come from? And more important, how do I find it?

Friends from my childhood went to church every Sunday and asked God for his help before bed, sleeping soundly because they knew all their prayers would be answered. They said grace at the table before meals, while I impatiently waited for the "Amen!" and could eat already. They sang songs about Jesus and how much he loved and cared for them.

Growing up Jew-ish (a.k.a. not super-religious), I learned the basics about Judaism in temple. I learned about Jewish culture and food. Food! Food! Food! I learned about our people's history and the Holocaust, which my grandparents and uncle had survived. I learned the Hebrew language for my bat mitzvah.

In my midteen years, I became a self-proclaimed

Jewddha (a hybrid Jew and Buddhist) and delved into the world of spirituality. I read *Be Here Now* by Ram Dass over and over, burned sage in my room (and sometimes accidentally through my carpet), and learned to count mala beads in a corduroy chair from the 1970s that I bought for twenty dollars at a thrift store. I didn't necessarily find God, but I did find something that felt like a hint of safety—a deep connection to something sturdier than I was. Somehow, though, I drifted away from the magnetic pull to spirituality before I would need it most.

When I was an adult and out in the real world, I had coworkers and friends with an abiding confidence that everything was happening in their lives perfectly (even when it seemed anything but). It was faith, I think. I watched them navigate challenges with ease, knowing God was working round the clock for them. I questioned often, but never out loud, how these people could fly on faith, believing some invisible man in the sky had their back. Because that's all I understood of what God was, or what he did. I wished I too could hand over the pressure of managing my failing, flailing life to someone or something else. If I could know God, he could surely help me with my shit show.

I wanted to believe that message everyone else around me was hearing: *God's got this. You can relax now.*

It was not long after that trip to Chicago that my

grandpa Leon—my dad's dad—said something to me in his last days of life. "I'm going to make sure you get better, even if I have to knock down God's door to do it," he croaked to me through the phone. And the first thought that came to my mind was, *How in the freakin' world does he believe in God?* Grandpa Leon had escaped the Nazis and built a bunker in the woods of Poland to save eighteen Jews from death. Grandpa Leon had seen almost his entire family be killed. Grandpa Leon had survived the Holocaust, but carried all the brutal memories with him when he left for the United States. He grew up believing in God, and not even all of *that* shook his resolve. He never blamed God for letting something so horrific happen, or started to doubt if God really existed in the first place. Perhaps his own survival only strengthened his conviction. Grandpa Leon, even in the face of humanity's greatest struggle, had mad faith. There were no *ifs* for him. Everything was going to work out. There was infinite order to everything, he seemed to know.

We humans like to prove to ourselves that there is good reason to believe something before we commit. But Grandpa Leon made me really question: What if we don't actually need to understand in order to believe? What if we don't need to make sense of every little detail before we take something on as truth and carry it forward? And what if faith only shows itself to us once we already believe?

It was then that I decided I would have faith. Just like that. Grandpa Leon was enough proof for me that faith was not only possible, but worth it. If he could have it, so could I. For me, maybe faith wasn't to be found in God, or any particular religion, but in believing in something bigger than me. I began to trust that some greater power, maybe even the entire Universe, had my back.

I am slightly disappointed that my faith seems to be wavering now in the midst of my epic Indian meltdown, although luckily I've learned that faith is fairly forgiving. It is not something that requires my constant attention and promise of loyalty. It often disappears, waiting for my call to it from desperate places like this, before it will come back and sustain me again. But, always, it returns.

"We are getting out of this hospital room, babe. Let's go see some cows!" my mom declares one late afternoon when I am hiding in bed, drowning in my own snot, sorrow, and self-pity—because, once again, I'm insatiably hungry, homesick, and can't stop crying. She is sitting next to me on the floor and has already offered all the things she always does when I'm a mess: tissues, hugs, and food (although there is not much to propose on the latter, we never stop trying).

That's how we end up walking around Delhi, with scarves wrapped around our faces to prevent us from coughing up sediment later. On cooler days, when people are trying to stay warm, the pollution is unrelenting, and the doctors warn us not to even go outside. We are still new at crossing these crazy erratic roads, so we hang on to each other tight when we do. If the situation looks extra-precarious, we do what a friend from home, a frequent visitor to India, taught us: find a friendly-looking local, grab an arm, and follow their expert lead to the other side. By the time we are a few blocks and ten minutes away from the hospital, we've seen three cows sitting in the street, two shoeless Indian children dancing in the traffic for money, a tuk-tuk overturned in front of a building, a mailman on a bicycle hurling the day's deliveries at front doors without stopping, and a chair salesman trying to shoo away a group of stray dogs fast asleep on his furniture. When I see my favorite grocery store, I light up. As much as I am inconvenienced by having to make my own teapot meals, I find some comfort in the normalcy of shopping. We walk in and I immediately begin rummaging through a giant disorganized shelf of food and paper products.

It is now, outside the hospital walls and energized by the world around me, that I recall a conversation I had with Dr. Shroff in the first days after my arrival.

At the request of one of the sisters, I had given the staff at Nutech a list of foods I could and could not eat. On the *could* list: protein and veggies. On the *could not* list: everything else. Over the past years, my brain has been programmed with messages like *dairy is bad because it causes inflammation*, *sugar feeds the Lyme bacteria*, and *carbs are evil*. And while maybe some of that has truth to it, being ridiculously strict about my diet only causes me more intense stress. And now, unstoppable hunger.

When Dr. Shroff saw the list, she came to my room with it and asked, "But what about your healthy cells? They need some sugar. Dairy is not bad for them. Carbs are okay in moderation! Each night, you can have a small amount of red wine and chocolate. You need some pleasure too." All I could think was, *Are you trying to kill me?*

It isn't until I am squatting on the mud-smudged grocery store floor that what she said begins to sink in. My whole existence for years now has been dedicated to "killing" Lyme. I have built my entire life around Lyme disease, the one thing that I *don't* want. What about the rest of me?

"Mom! Look!" I scream as I hold up a box of Kraft mac and cheese that was wedged between a bag of lentils and a box of basmati rice.

"Oh my Gaaaaawd, babe!" She runs over in disbelief. I keep digging and soon find a packaged chocolate lava cake, the kind where you add hot water to the plastic tray full of batter and it magically puffs up into dessert. It's inflatable chocolate cake, and it's a frickin' miracle! Where is the genie granting me these wishes? There is nothing

GMO-free, organic, or natural about this food jackpot, but I am thrilled!

Clutching these boxes as if they are solid gold, I rush them to the register and pay a total of 200 rupees, or three American dollars. I have only a tiny bit of guilt about the quality of this food, but even that will be obsolete soon. The perspective I am about to gain is priceless.

What if, in my furious effort to find the cure, I have been missing something critically important all along? There is no question that I need these stem cells to work for me. There is no debate that I need my legs and my health back. And no one would argue that I also need to stop bursting into tears and get my act together. But until that happens, what if I also need something that has been completely within my reach all along? My own permission to save myself any way I can. What if I loosen the death grip I have on my own life? What if true faith means grabbing on to whatever you can in each moment, and letting that be enough to carry you on? What if there are a hundred opportunities to save your life every single day? And none of them look like *the cure*, but actually are essential fragments of it. What if everything that came before now did not seem like healing, but was a tiny step toward it? And what if today, when I can't change any of my circumstances, I can save a little piece of myself WITH THIS INFLATABLE CHOCOLATE CAKE?

After dropping Mom off at the bed-and-breakfast, I go back to my hospital room, boil the kettle, pour water into the plastic dish, and seal the lid back on quickly. I think of Zach and our favorite ritual—pretending it's his birthday on just any random Tuesday. We bake a cake, pour the entire container of sprinkles on it, light the candles, then giggle through a verse of "For he's a jolly good fellow" before making as many wishes as we want. There are no rules in our world, especially on fake birthdays.

When four minutes have passed, I uncover the container with care. I scoop each bite out of the tray, moving it slowly to my mouth and savoring it, as if Julia Child has prepared it especially for me. Some food is good for your body, but this food is good for my soul. With every rich chocolate morsel, I sink deeper into the faith that somehow, I will be okay. Maybe, hopefully, even better than that.

Sitting on my bed, full of the best unhealthy thing I've eaten in a very long time, I hear a man with a strong, low voice calling out in Hindi from the back alley behind the hospital. The voice is moving, waxing and waning, amplified by a megaphone. I can't understand what he's saying, perhaps a prayer of some kind, but the rich tone soothes me. I peer out the side window of my room, but can't spot him. I imagine him as a gray-haired, white-robed guru on a slow-moving bicycle, weaving through people and cows to deliver his message. God on a loudspeaker, maybe.

I grab my *Hidden Messages in Water* book and ask into thin air: *What do I need to know in this moment? Please say it's that this all might be turning around for me.*

I flip to a random page for a sign and see the striking images—groundwater before and after an earthquake in the western part of Japan's Honshu Island. Immediately before the earthquake, no crystals were formed, as if the water sensed the impending doom. But after the earth's rumble, ah! Once some time had passed, the ability of the water to form crystals returned yet again.

Yes, the truest kind of healing comes from the quake that causes the cracks.

4

Pierced

"Babe, I want to get my nose pierced like the Indians!" my mom announces excitedly out of the blue.

We are strolling down the main drag in the hub of our neighborhood when she drops this bombshell. It is a brisk and bright afternoon and the smog is unusually absent. I have just purchased my usual two marigold garlands from a woman selling them off a fuzzy blanket on the sidewalk. These garlands, called *varmala*, have an unpleasant smell—a little bit like rotting fruit—but I can't stop buying them! The fluffy pom-pom suns, strung like necklaces, brighten the whole street and my hospital room. We visit this area of Green Park almost daily now, and it's starting to feel like any Main Street in America to us. We know which shop to visit for the best Indian sweets—multicolored glutinous gifts, made with rich flavors of sweet syrup, cardamom, saffron, and mango. We've also discovered a coffee shop with the perfect cup of chai. It has a cozy bookstore in the back with a great variety of Indian books, some of which are in English. We feel worldly and cultured when we shop there. I sink into my chai and a book called *Q & A*, which will later become the blockbuster movie *Slumdog Millionaire*. Mom always gets a latte, which tastes like those at home but is made with soya milk, and another Nicholas Sparks book. She's going through them both at record rates. We have a book exchange at the hospital, and Nicholas Sparks books are a hot commodity.

"Will you do it with me? We can have matching piercings!" my sixty-two-year-old mother asks.

Something is happening to my mom in India. She is not typically conservative by any means, but here, she is more carefree than I've ever seen her. India has brought out her inner flower child and she seems to be fully embracing it. In this crazy city, she is automatically 10 percent more fun, willing, and even a little bit wild.

I think this is true about me too. What I love about travel is how you can and will do things you'd never do at home. There is a freedom of some sort that cannot be captured in your typical environment. Something about being away from home makes the not-normally-okay somehow okay. The rules of home fade across borders, perhaps because no one is keeping score—not even me. The order of daily life is absent, and therefore all my inclinations to adhere to it are as well. Here, it's all YOLO (*you only live once*), all the time.

"Come on, babe, I came all the way to India for you," Mom jokes—or maybe it's not a joke. Her head is tilted to the side and her ponytail is swinging with hope.

"Let's do it!" I agree, rolling my eyes with a playful smile.

We walk only a few blocks before spotting a fancy-shmancy jewelry shop.

"Over there." I point, already embracing the adventure. There is an armed guard outside and gold chains hanging in the window.

We enter the store and I approach the suited man behind the counter to ask if they do nose piercings.

"Ahh, yes, suuuuure," he says, making no eye contact, but sizing up our noses from a few feet away. He claps in the air and a barefoot teenager appears from the back room almost instantly. His hair is growing in all different directions and his shirt is torn. In his hands, he holds a pair of rusty pliers, a little container of jewelry, a blue pen, cotton balls, and a canister of alcohol. I guess he is the piercer.

"You're first," I say to my mom, caught somewhere in

between a *this is stupid* and a *this is hilarious* laugh. I should stop us both from letting a shoeless stranger put permanent holes in our faces, but it's too entertaining. Mom sits down on the stool and closes her eyes, and the boy puts a blue pen mark on her left nostril. Women in India are always pierced on the left side of the nose. According to Hinduism, this is one way to honor Parvathi, the goddess of marriage. A large nose ring, joined from the nose to the ear with a chain, is an integral part of bridal jewelry. It is also said that the left side corresponds with the reproductive system in women, so the piercing allegedly reduces pain during childbirth. Some also say it can alleviate endometriosis, a painful condition where the uterine lining grows on other parts of the reproductive system. This is another disease on my never-ending list. Since I first got my period at thirteen, I've had several surgeries to ease my agonizing and heavy menstrual cycles. None of them have worked. Maybe this is my ticket to monthly serenity. No pressure, piercing guru!

There is no consult or pleasantries before he lines up a long, thin needle to Mom's nose. He never asks about her preference for sides, but I don't think she cares. She is fidgeting in her seat with anticipation. I'm the nervous mom here and she's the excited teenager. Capturing the entire thing on video, I watch through the camera. When the boy makes the puncture, her only reaction is a slow,

tight blink of her eyes. She says nothing and is done before she can even tear up. He removes the needle, inserts a
thin gold rod, and pushes it through. Bending the piece of
metal into a hoop, he finishes and then tips his chin up for
her to get out of the seat.

"Woweee, I love it!" she says, admiring herself in the
mirror.

The piercer doesn't speak English, but when he sees
my mom standing proud in all her boldness and bejeweled
glory, he finally cracks a smile.

He waves me over to brave the stool next. It is with my
butt in the seat that I feel the weight of what a truly stupid
idea this could be. My immune system can't even handle
a cold, let alone an infection from a piercing gone wrong.
I glance down at my right hand, which has an IV line inserted and taped down. I cover it with my left hand as if
to shield it from seeing this irresponsible act. The piercing
hurts more than I imagined but not enough to make me
cry. I move to touch my nose gently when it's over, as confirmation that I really did it, but the boy swats me away.
The man behind the counter claps once more, and the boy
leaves as quickly as he appeared.

We pay about twenty American dollars and are free to
go. Pierced and high on our impulsive decision, we leave
the shop—two schoolgirls who have just taken their parents' car without asking.

"What do you think the other kids will say?" Mom asks curiously as we walk back toward the hospital.

"Lauren will hate it," I reply confidently, because my sister is the most straitlaced of our bunch and would definitely file this under *what were you thinking?* "David won't care at all," I predict, because he is both super laid-back *and* a serious mama's boy. She does no wrong in his eyes.

"And what about Dad?" she questions next.

"He'll totally love it!" I assure her. My dad loves everything about her and I don't think this will be any exception. I adore how my parents let each other be who they are. They don't drag each other to activities the other one wouldn't enjoy, never get mad or jealous if one does something fun without the other, and don't ask each other for permission to be themselves.

I fleetingly wonder what Jay would think about this new addition to my face. What I do with my nose and my life is no longer any of his business, but I still find myself tangled in the aftermath of our complicated love.

I learned early on that Jay and I worked best when we were floating blissfully in the whirlwind of us. Even before I got sick and the days of partying and fun were long gone, I began to see that our love was built in a bubble. While we did epically better than I might have predicted if I'd known what was to come, I saw that when stressful forces shook our world—an issue at work, a family strain, even just a fight with each other—we splintered a little. I made it my job to compartmentalize feelings, thoughts, and even my relationships with other people to protect our chamber of happiness.

There were times when Jay drank a lot, especially after I got sick. And these were the times he'd sometimes become resentful, jealous, or unhappy with me for any little reason. And by this time, I had transferred my sensitivity about upsetting my parents to my fear of upsetting Jay. I developed a persistent case of it's-my-fault syndrome, believing when he was upset or in an off mood, it had to be because of me. I jumped to overcompensate for tensions in our relationship. "I know you don't mean it," I'd say when he said hurtful things to me. When he didn't come home or call as promised, I'd reassure him: "I know this isn't you." I ran to excuse him, to take blame, to save him from himself—and from breaking my heart.

Would Jay think this piercing was a cool and independent move, or would he be irritated that I'd done something cool and independent without him? Even now, ten thousand miles away, I am still hard at work in my head wondering what would make him happy.

It was about a year into our romance, just as the novelty of my cool bleached-blond hair was wearing off and my liver was tiring from all the booze, that I started to see how tugged and torn I was between the real *me* and the *me* that fit best with Jay.

"I don't feel like drinking today," I said one Sunday afternoon, as we got ready to go to Mike and Mallory's house for a barbecue. Mike and Mallory are a kind, mellow couple, Jay's longtime friends—who were always with a cocktail in one hand and a joint in the other.

"You're just not as fun when you don't drink," Jay replied quickly, as if he'd been waiting to tell me this forever.

Crushed, I cheerfully consoled him. "I will totally have fun even if I don't feel like drinking."

"It's not the same," he rebutted.

"Okay, maybe I'll have a couple of drinks," I compromised, and off we went to Mike and Mallory's in a car stuffed with silence.

"What's up?" Mallory asked me in the kitchen as soon as we got a second alone.

I could confide in Mallory, because even though she was friends with Jay first, she was always on my team.

"I'm not fun when I don't drink," I shared. I turned my head in Jay's direction as he chatted with Mike. Mallory flipped her ash-colored bangs into the air with the breath from her hearty laugh.

That day, each time my glass was empty, Mallory

grabbed it from me and brought it to the drink station she had set up in the kitchen. I saw her refill my cup six different times: lemonade only, no vodka.

I kept chugging.

On the patio later, Jay leaned into my stone-cold sober body with a lit cigarette and whispered, "You are so much fun tonight! See why I love it when you drink?"

When I went inside the house, I mouthed in wide words to a totally baked Mallory, "Thaaank yooouuu." She nodded back and winked, exhaling from her pipe.

This story is both small and insignificant, and also everything. Because it would repeat itself over and over in so many different ways. This story represents a million things that I ignored in our relationship, a million things that, had I listened to them, would have made my life difficult while I was busy forcing it to go smoothly. This is a story I'll never forget, a story that will come into my mind often when I try to push away the things I'm noticing about my life. The world is always telling us stories about who it thinks we should be. But it's up to us to know and own our own truth.

On that day, for whatever reason, I recognized that Mallory's story was the same truth my heart was trying to speak to me: *I am good enough just how I am.* For the record, I am also a damn good time on pink lemonade.

I can feel that truth today, pierced right through my nose. I feel a little bit out of character, but I'm also surprised by how *me* it actually feels.

When Mom and I return to the hospital, my dad is where we left him, carefully studying the user's manual for his new Indian alarm clock. He looks up from his inch-thick magnifying glass and notices our gold-adorned noses.

"Where'd you get *that*?" he asks, his eyes glistening toward my mom. But before we can answer, he lifts his hands to the air in disbelief and confirms what we already knew. "It's really fucking awesome!" My dad never left the sixties. He raised us on Carole King, Paul Simon, and James Taylor. Peace, love, and fun are his religion. At this moment, we are shining examples of his spirit, and it's no secret he is totally loving it.

In India, I may be coming undone, but I am also becoming unclenched.

In these past few weeks, I have started to suspect that life cannot be manhandled and things cannot be perfect. No matter how hard I try to force them, I cannot be anything close to the vision of my strongest, most pulled-together self. And because of this, I feel the urge to stop trying so hard—something that is impossible for me at home. In this erratic and free-for-all country, it is becoming clear what the crushing pressure of holding on so tight has done to me. Not only has it made my life harder than it needs to be, but I start to really wonder how much this pattern has affected my body too. What is the cost of clinging to stability and consistency?

Up to now, I have tried to control everything and have ended up sick, in a foreign country, and battling for my health. While I suppose it could be worse (or maybe not), let's face it: my regimen of control may possibly not be the most effective approach to life. I think it's time to let go.

When I decide I am ready to start letting go, I recognize that I don't even fully know what *letting go* means, because I am such an expert at *holding on*.

I hold on to fear about my body and my future.

I hold buckets of resentment from my past.

I hold frustration and bitterness because there was no cure for me at home.

I hold on to relationships with people whom I let tell me who I am.

I hold on to grudges like they are gems that will one day make me rich.

I hold tight to the idea of how I think things should be.

I hold myself to impossible standards, responsible for everything and everyone.

I decide to define *letting go* as going with the flow of life instead of fighting it. I will no longer try to manipulate the unchangeable. I will not swim upstream, against the current, like the one stupid fish in the river going the wrong way, the hard way. I'm pretty sure I've been *that* fish.

It seems there is no better place to try this than in the magical, glorious chaos of India. If I can conquer letting go here, I can conquer it anywhere.

From now on, here's the deal I make with myself. If it won't kill me to go with the flow, I will. And if I can't let go, I will accept the horrendous feeling of being dragged—the emotional torment of trying to wrestle with what is beyond my control, like time, space, my dislike for *saag paneer*, traffic jams all damn day, air I can't breathe without choking, and wherever the Universe is intent on taking me.

When I first begin this experiment of letting go, I'll fail quite a few times, only to rein my efforts back in like a cowboy who temporarily lost the lead on his horse. *Let go, it's okay. Let go.* Then, *No no no, you idiot! Fight!* Then again, *Let go.* Each time I feel resistance rising within me, I remind myself of my two choices—let go on my own or be dragged. Soon it feels like letting go is almost always the better option.

When I find myself resenting the beeping horns outside, I decide to lean into them. I study the traffic, observing carefully to see what they are honking about. I am fascinated to find that all the honking is actually a language: instead of using blinkers to indicate their next move, drivers beep before they change lanes and even when they are saying thank you to another driver for letting them merge. This does not immediately make me a fan of the *beep beep beeps*, but it makes me part of the game instead of an enemy of it.

When I see Dr. Shroff in physio and she asks me the usual "How are you?" I start to panic. I want to run away, preempting an attack on whatever she thinks I am doing wrong. When I decide to let go and speak the truth—that some things are good and some are not—she tells me to focus on the good, that I can heal myself, and that I must let go of all thoughts that are not working for me. "I'm trying!" I agree genuinely and with a smile. This is the first time I feel her words not as criticism, but as a message with some kind of truth. There is a new softness in our exchange. She even notices the nose ring and tells me it's cute. I think we are making progress. Maybe.

I press on, proud of my successes, making a brand-new conscious decision in each moment: to turn away from the fight within me . . . and *let go*.

I do it each evening when the sister comes to do my IV and doesn't use the disinfecting protocol that the nurses at home would. *Let go.* I make the decision when the tuk-tuk driver promises he knows where he's going and then loops around the city for two hours because he clearly doesn't.

Let go. I make the decision when I see the hospital's "premier dry-cleaning service provider" set up on the street corner, hanging my delicates from a makeshift clothesline, then beating them with a wooden stick for all the world to see and all the city's dust to cling to. Now I know why my laundry has been returning with holes. *Let go.* It is really not long before I learn that letting go won't kill me and I start to enjoy it.

And that's how I end up packed into a car with my parents and our bags on a winter road trip to Agra—the famous city in the northern state of Uttar Pradesh, and home to the Taj Mahal. Because there is nothing that throws you out of your comfort zone more than agreeing to head off into the great wild of India for a four-hour drive with a stranger behind the wheel.

My parents have been gently cheerleading, asking me to consider a trip outside the city's perimeter. Up until now, I have been too worried about how I'd feel, what I'd eat, and being in the car for so long while I'm so emotionally unsteady. But it is now, after three weeks of keeping company with the most unstable version of myself I've ever known, and surviving it, that I have agreed to visit the magnificent spiritual mecca of the Taj Mahal.

Dr. Shroff has approved me to leave overnight. "Good! You will not focus on illness there," she tells me.

"True!" I reply, with sincerity that matches hers.

Most of the patients here have already made the journey to the Taj and have told us we must see it. "You can't go to India and not see the Taj Mahal!" "It's only four hours away. How could you not?" "It's unimaginable, you'll see. This is a once-in-a-lifetime chance." I am a total antitourist, typically avoiding these types of excursions like the plague, but I am also desperate to flee Delhi.

Carpe diem!

The ride to Agra, home to the beloved and spiritually magnetic mausoleum, is rough and rugged, like all car journeys here. It feels like there is no asphalt beneath our wheels and we are simply being dragged over rocks and potholes toward our destination.

Our English-speaking driver, Raj, chats in his thick, melodious accent most of the way. Raj is well educated, but tells us that unless he has enough money to bribe someone in India, he cannot get a good job.

"If only I could buy a car instead of working for someone else," he declares, "I would be reeeech!" But with the tiny salary he gets, there is just no way to get ahead. "Your America truly theee laaand of opportunity!"

Driving past the government officials' mansions, which look like they are located in the Beverly Hills of Delhi, he points a finger out the window and says, "Theeese are the homes of the corruption leaders." He doesn't crack a smile.

I am absorbing the sights and sounds from the window

in awe, camera in hand, trying to capture the things that fly by too quickly. Dad is in the front seat doing the same, and my mom is in the back with me, peering out the window in wonder. In between capturing shots of wild boars running, children dancing, and men pushing food carts of every kind, I use the technique I've learned to avoid getting carsick in India: look out the side window, only and always. When I've looked through the front window here, I want to jump out and walk, convinced it's the only way to arrive at my destination alive.

During every car ride, you are guaranteed to come face-to-face with cows s-l-o-w-l-y crossing the road, causing the driver to terrifyingly swerve with no warning; cars skidding into oncoming traffic to make a left turn; people running in front of your taxi to sell you a calendar in Hindi, or a single carrot; and a host of other absurdities. If you ever visit this hectic, amazing country, simply focus on one thing when traveling by car: side window only.

One of the towns we pass through looks as if it is made from nothing but brightly dyed trash. It appears that a bomb has exploded, scattering a sea of rainbow candy wrappers. Animals and children play among the piles of rubbish as if they are there for the purpose of pure enjoyment. People are drinking from puddles of water outside their huts, which are made of mud and sugarcane. Kids are playing naked. People living along the sides of this stretch of road to Agra have no money to eat and are drinking and bathing in filthy water, but have goats that seem to be worth a fortune. The furry friends are lovingly decked out in sweaters, bells, and jewels.

This would be the mother of all MasterCard commercials:

Bottled drinking water: $1
Enough rice to last a week: $6
Making your goat's wardrobe a priority: PRICELESS

We arrive at the Taj just in time to see several phases of the sunset in its last hour before dusk. Raj parks and shows us where we go next, to meet our already-assigned tour guide. Cars and buses are not allowed to come within five hundred meters of the entrance. This prevents vehicle exhaust from tarnishing the building.

The rush to enter the glorious Taj Mahal is like trying to get into Boston's Fenway Park—everyone is crammed in line to get to the front first, only to go nowhere at the same time.

Men in one line and women in another, we are patted down and our bags are lazily searched, with the guards often looking in another direction while they do their rummaging. My backpack is full of pill bottles, tubes of lip moisturizer, and the single roll of toilet paper I carry everywhere after learning the hard way that some venues in India are BYOTP.

Once we are declared weapon-or-whatever-free, we flood through the entrance and get our first glimpse of the opulent architectural icon. Beyond the sprawling garden and grand fountain that opens before us, we see the Taj Mahal, meaning Crown of the Palace, standing at a towering 240 feet. It is made entirely of ornately carved, glistening white marble. There are four huge pillars that encircle the Taj and appear to be protectors, the keepers of this marvelous palatial structure. The pillars are tipped away from the dome ever so slightly, constructed this way so the tomb would be saved if they were ever to crumble.

Inside the gates, the race begins for photo opportunities. It is a sea of cameras, bobbing heads hidden behind them.

We see a sign with our name on it and wave to our tour guide.

"Hello! Ready for photo?" he asks, and escorts us over to get the best shots. We fall into pose quickly for our family photo at the freakin' Taj Mahal in India!

"This Taj was built for Mughal Emperor Shah Jahan's favorite wife!" our guide explains, swinging his hand up in a circular motion toward it. I immediately snub my nose at this whole "favorite wife" thing, until I learn that the emperor had it built for her as a tomb, after she died during the birth of their fourteenth child. Any woman who had that many children deserved to be the "favorite." It turns out she was the third *and* the favorite. But I do wonder if he told all his wives that.

We wander around for quite a while, our shoes hiding under the required cotton covers that protect the gardens and the ground of this forty-two-acre complex. I never realized how massive the entire area would be. I am going slowly, at a turtle's pace, because that's the only way I can keep up right now. But I am still going.

Mom and Dad are spaced generously around me. It is now that I feel something I have not felt in quite a while: the ease of my parents. Through the past years, I have been acutely aware of their worry, their cautionary observation of me when they think I might be in pain or discomfort. But right now, I am once again their little girl, and they are just regular parents able to enjoy a new family adventure.

As we continue our stroll through the grounds and toward the Taj, we see women draped in saris sitting on the lawns, little lime-green parrots perched in trees, and photographers getting the shots of a lifetime. The closer we get, the more impressive the massiveness of the building becomes. Over a thousand elephants were used to carry materials here from all over the world. The white marble from Rajasthan is what the Taj is most recognized for, but the different stones that are inset in the marble is what gives it life: jade, crystal, turquoise, jasper, lapis lazuli, sapphire, and carnelian. It took decades to complete this masterpiece. It looks like it would take no less.

When we finally get right up to the building that holds the tomb, we've been wandering around for at least forty-five minutes. I reach my hand out and the wall feels cool, like a bathroom tile floor first thing in the morning. The calligraphy inscribed on the surface of the Taj Mahal is remarkable, consisting mostly of verses and prayers from the holy Quran. To see the marble-carved floral imagery so close-up is to study the petals of a flower held gently in your hand after seeing the entire garden only from a distance.

The crowds that pile into the actual structure holding the tomb are packed like herds of sheep, only less polite. Our guide asks if we want to enter.

"You can enter, but I give warning," he says, holding his hand out as a stop sign. "Your white skin may be appealing to others and therefore it's possible it is dangerous! It's best you don't go in such tight quarters where you may be groped."

"We're gonna skip it!" Dad cuts in immediately, Mom and I nodding with utter approval. Getting felt up in a tomb would be wrong on so many levels.

After a few hours, I am pleased to be able to still be walking around, high on the validity of being part of thousands of culturally mature people who flock to the Taj each year. I feel like a champ for lasting this long and with less pain than expected; the continuous deep throbbing still exists inside, but it is no longer overpowering all of me.

As my physical pain becomes less of a focus, I am present in ways I've never been before. I notice blackbirds are screaming, flying high circles in the sky. I stop for long moments to take them in, listening to the *click-click* of Dad's camera as he follows their flight. The breeze that blows my hair into my face feels sharp on my cheek. My awareness of my surroundings is heightened and I have less of an obsession about my body and what it is or isn't doing. I am fully, and only, right where I am. I recognize this awareness as something I learned from studying Buddhism. I've tried to achieve it many times in my life, but especially since coping with physical pain and illness—this mindfulness of my current state, without being attached to it. At home, it's always seemed unattainable. But in India, I am a natural wanderer, a drifter at heart, and able to be present without having to strive greatly for it. Although I am a Virgo to the core, often craving order, analysis, organization, and direction, there is a part of me deep inside that needs none of that. I need only to *be*. And that part of me seems to have a surprising and direct connection to total and pure joy. When away from home and my ideas of what should or shouldn't be, it turns out, I do not freak out. Well, not always. Instead, I open up. I slow down. I give myself the permission to be free, to pay attention to what is right in front of me. Everything is new and vibrant, pulling me toward it.

The night is dark when we make our way toward the exit, and as we walk, I inhale the pure awesomeness of each step. There is no agenda in these quieter moments of my journey, no need for an urgent cure, and no immediate awareness of or thoughts about the stem cell treatment I came for.

Instead, I sense an unconscious, unprompted internal shift. Particles of my old self are being left behind on these cherished grounds. I do not have all the answers to who I am today, in these precious slivers of time. In fact, I am not even entirely aware how precious they are. But one thing is undeniably true: I am no longer willing to be the girl who holds on so tight that she breaks her own spirit to do it. *Let go. Let go. Let go.*

Under the remarkable towering marble and the black sky scattered with stars, the things that make me feel most alive become thoroughly clear: the glow on the crescent moon above me, the spark of a tiny new part of myself, and the brilliance of having a picture with my parents at one of the greatest destinations on earth. *When life blows*, I think, *may I always return effortlessly to this day.*

5

To Begin Again

WEEK FOUR

Party big or go home. This is the mood that welcomes us back from our trip to the Taj. The hospital, like the entire city, is an explosion of decorations, music, and festivities in preparation for Christmas and New Year's Eve. Holiday spirit is in full swing.

I am awakened at 7 a.m. on the last Saturday morning of 2007 to the hammering and clanking of poles. Thanks to the rat, who is still winning, I continue to sleep in the empty room next door to mine. But there is no view from here, so I can't figure out what all the commotion is about. I shuffle my way back to "our" room, where I can see out to the front of the building and all the action.

When I peep out the window with my squinty, swollen eyes, I see full-on party prep for tonight's celebration unfolding on the front patio and sidewalk. Typically, things happen at a snail's pace in Delhi. On the neighboring building, it's taken six men two weeks to paint one wall; but this morning, outside the hospital, three workers have hoisted up tents, stages, decorations, and music equipment as if they were simply rolling out a Slip 'N Slide. If I hadn't just heard the noise myself, I would have assumed it was unfurled with gusto overnight by magic elves.

It is still the very early hours of the day when, out of nowhere, Susan from across the hall jumps through my doorway. "Justin on the third floor just peed for the first time on his own!" she yells, running out before I can match her excitement. She has just heard this news from *her* neighbor, and it's my job to keep it going.

"Justin peed!" I shout to my direct neighbor, and hear it echoing down the corridor in a morning chorus: "Justin peeed! . . . Justin peeed! . . . Justin peeed! . . ."

Justin is a twenty-five-year-old from Texas who was paralyzed in a tractor accident. For a paraplegic, being able to use his bladder on his own again is a huge accomplishment—one that most of us take for granted.

But Justin is not the only one who is starting the day with a bang.

Chavi's face reads *HAPPY* from across the room when I arrive for my morning physio session. It seems that the hospital is abuzz with good news.

Mike, who is fifty years old and suffers from an extremely rare muscle disease (so rare that the chance of getting it is literally one in a million), has just received the news of a 20 percent improvement in his latest muscle enzyme test. With the help of stem cells, his body is reversing muscle deterioration.

Ravi, a one-year-old Indian boy with cerebral palsy, has never been able to make eye contact or reach for things on his own. Today he is proudly and successfully reaching for colored blocks. The whole room cheers him on as he drops them, one by one, with great determination and perfect hand-eye coordination, into an empty fishbowl.

When I finally make it over to Chavi, who is waiting by an empty physio bed, she is beaming. "Tonight will be your first big Indian holiday bash! You are going to really love it!"

Everyone is high on thrills today.

We have just increased my physio sessions to twice a day and have added Velcro strap-on weights to my arms and legs. Physio is getting less challenging because I'm getting stronger, but more challenging because Chavi keeps upping the ante. But since today is a celebration, we'll all be let out of school early—only one physio session. Par-tay!

"This is the coldest snap in Delhi in nearly six years!" Chavi says, fake-shivering to make a point as she moves and stretches my calves on the table. She is bundled up in a jacket and two scarves, because it's forty-eight degrees out-side. Winter in Delhi starts in late November and peaks in January, with average temperatures around fifty-five de-grees Fahrenheit. For the rest of the year, the city is sti-fling hot. Delhiites don't adapt to this chill very well. The cold weather doesn't compare to a New York City winter, but it is a big deal to them. Every night, the sisters bunch together in the nursing stations, wrap themselves in blan-kets, and cozy up to flasks of hot chai.

"Ooh my, your thighs have grown!" Chavi shrieks while using her pocket-size measuring tape. "Can you tell you have firmed?!" she asks me, grinning eagerly.

"Yes, I can, thank you," I mouth in a whisper, signaling to her that we don't have to share my increased thigh size with the entire room. I love Chavi's enthusiasm, but this is not group news in my opinion.

"Very thick and good!" she says, slapping them once more for good measure.

Although my many balancing tricks in physio don't prove perfection yet, I haven't tripped in weeks. Some days, when I try to walk along the tiled line on the physio room floor, one foot in front of another, I do it so well that I'd feel just as safe if I were on a tightrope. Other days, I am very thankful that Chavi is standing by my side to catch me when I fall. If Johnny Cash only knew how many times I hum his "I Walk the Line" in a single day.

My family arrives to the evening holiday party with excitement, but no particular expectation. Mom and I have hands covered in *mehndi*, intricate designs created from the powdered leaves of the henna plant. The markets are often dotted with artists offering books full of these gorgeous patterns to choose from. While mehndi was originally only applied on the palms, it now most often covers the hands and feet, and sometimes backs and shoulders. Traditional designs are created from representations of the sun and are typically applied for Hindu weddings and festivals. "We liiiiike!" Sahana says as the spokesperson for the group of sisters who greet us at the party.

The lobby is packed with folding chairs, wheelchairs, hospital staff, and patients and their families. About twenty locals outside have noticed the commotion and press their faces up against the large windows to look in.

The evening's party begins with a form of classical dance called Bharatanatyam, originating in the Hindu temples of the South Indian state of Tamil Nadu. The name of the dance is formed by combining the words *bharata* and *natyam*, which translate loosely to *dance* and *emotion*.

The dancers are wearing gorgeous saris in splendid purples and deep reds, with pleats that fall in the front coming down from the waist. They move perfectly to the band's music. When they twirl and twist, the saris widen like paper hand fans. Their henna-tattooed feet only highlight their fancy footwork. Gorgeous jeweled headpieces sit like crowns on their heads and flowers look to be blooming from their hair. The women's faces are painted with bold makeup, totally captivating us with constantly changing expressions that capture the mood of each moment.

This party is full-on Bollywood-style, and everyone is loving the treat.

When the dance is over, Dr. Shroff grabs the mic to make an announcement about the special meal waiting for us. She points toward the buffet-style tables outside.

"We have the authentic meal . . . and also the non-spicy for the wimps." She seems uncomfortable being in the spotlight as she laughs with her dainty giggle.

A few minutes later, she approaches me outside where I am trying both the food for wimps *and* the authentic food (gasp!). Dad is at a table nearby chatting to the doctors. Mom has linked arms with the dancers as if they're about to do the cancan, having her picture taken like she's one of the girls.

"Are you sure you don't want to try the Indian food for daily meals?" Dr. Shroff asks, using the moment wisely. She has not forgotten the food drama of late. "You may begin to like it with an open mind! Look! You are eating it already."

Let go, I think, before I can muster up any resistance to

this idea. I'm not sure if I'm tricking myself, but I actually feel my body *wants* this food.

"I think it's a great idea," I reply, grinning and proud of myself. "Thank you."

The party is finally winding down when I hear my dad's voice on the loudspeaker system. He and the daughter of another patient have gotten hold of the band's microphone and are performing a rookie rendition of James Blunt's "You're Beautiful." They are taking turns pointing and singing to each person left sitting in the folding chairs. This is karaoke at its worst, but everyone is having a blast. My dad was born to be an entertainer. He was the annual Santa Claus at the local nursing home in our hometown, dressed up as Elvis for his Vegas-themed fortieth birthday party, and is the enthusiastic joke-teller of any group when he can steal the floor.

When I get back to my room after the party is really finished (it's not over till my dad sings, apparently), I receive an unexpected evening surprise.

The sisters arrive to tell me that I am getting an especially large IV infusion of stem cells tonight. "We begin to increase your dose tonight! Every ten days you will receive large amount," one of them explains, shaking the glass bottle in front of me. This is huge compared to the typical small shot in my thigh or arm. This is a *mega*dose.

Sahana hangs the bottle with stem cells and saline by

my bed and hooks me up to it. For the twenty minutes it takes to infuse, I visualize the cells like glitter in a snow globe, lighting up my body. I enjoy every minute, eyes closed, my iPod serenading me with Smokey Robinson songs to drown out the rest of the world.

Two hours later, I have a horrific feverish feeling and body aches so severe they feel like spasms. Stabbing pains in my toes are shooting up through my legs at double the intensity they normally do. Every inch of me feels like it is throwing an urgent fit. Sweat is gushing out of me. I call for Sahana and she immediately summons Dr. Ashish.

"This is fantastic!" he says with excitement. "Your sleepy immune system is waking up! We are also correcting your nervous system. The large concentration of cells circulating through your body in a very short period of time has a stimulating effect. This is the repair work!" He is ecstatic that I am in bed, in a fetal position, pleading for relief.

This is not the first time I've been in this position, and it's also not the first time a doctor has rejoiced over it.

It was 2005 when I got my first really terrible diagnosis—the diagnosis that would kick off the worst years of my life. The ones that came before it seemed hardly anything compared to *this* one. I had just turned twenty-five years old.

Even though my late teens and early twenties hadn't afforded me perfect health, I always thought physical symptoms from one thing or another were just a part of life. In the years before the Puerto Vallarta trip with Jay, when the pain struck my legs, I had seen my doctor for various complaints: migraines, waves of random nausea, problematic periods, unexplained fatigue, a case of shingles, and a flu that lingered for months. But these were things that he described as "maybe hormones" and "probably nothing."

Jay and I had just gotten back from Mexico and I returned to work at Harley-Davidson, the icon of freedom, stuck not only in my cubicle but in my declining body as well. My job sounded glamorous, but I was secretly most attached to my title of marketing director and not the job itself. I told everyone how much I loved it when they asked. "It's so fun! It's great!" I'd say. But the reality was that my car reeked of leather from carting jackets and chaps to events, I worked almost every weekend, and my boss was the human version of autocorrect. Whatever I did or said, she'd steamroll it with whatever *she* thought I should do or say. I stayed out of her view, hidden away in my corner overflowing with flyers for specials we were running. I was trying to ignore how much I hated my job and how my legs were failing me—always in pain, weak, and causing me to trip when I walked. I was also trying to ignore that even though I was in love with Jay, the fractures that had already started were only getting deeper. Still, I pressed on. I treated it all like I treated my credit card bills. *Ignore and it does not exist. Nothing to see here.*

That's when my feet and legs started tingling. A brand-new symptom. This was when I knew that whatever had happened in Mexico was definitely not a fluke. Even a twenty-five-year-old knows that tingling is not "hormones" or "nothing."

A month later, when I finally made it to the neurologist, I was that girl begging her boyfriend to cut her legs off.

Dr. Ourm, a gentle man with a thick Persian accent, did several tests that involved sticking needles in my legs and measuring the electrical activity of my nerves. And when he was done, he explained that my body was eating away at the covering of my own nerves, called the myelin sheath. I had a disease called chronic inflammatory demyelinating polyneuropathy, CIDP for short; and it was going to take a lot, he told me, to try to stop it.

This is the kind of diagnosis that turns your normal life into an out-of-control, spiraling mess. This is the kind of diagnosis that takes you from the person who knows nothing about your body and how it functions to the person who has to know *everything*. This is the kind of diagnosis that heaves you hard and fast into a whole new world—of medical terms, merciless insurance companies, and statistics—ready or not, here you come. Published reports estimate that as few as 1 in 100,000 people have CIDP, this type of neuropathy caused by an autoimmune reaction.

"I'll fill out the disability papers. You're not going back to work, Amy," Dr. Ourm said to me.

"But I have to be back after lunch," I argued.

Dr. Ourm knew what was coming.

At each follow-up visit, he would show me a laminated pain chart, a line of smiley faces from happy to sad, and numbers from one to ten. Number one on the chart, accompanied by a very chipper smiley face, meant you were in only a small amount of pain. Number ten, accompanied by an overdramatic sad face, meant you were living in misery. That ten was me, almost always, despite strong medications, including handfuls of narcotic painkillers each day.

That pain chart became the gauge for my day-to-day life, and provided a much-needed lighthearted game for Jay and me.

Jay would wake up in the morning and say, "Good morning, honey. I'm a two today. And you?" I'd often reply with something like "I was up with a nine all night, but I'm feeling a bit better now. I am hoping one day I can be a two like you!"

But I never became a two; not even close.

After months of no improvement, Dr. Ourm had a possible solution. He offered me an experimental treatment with great promise, called intravenous immunoglobulin, or IVIG. Ironically, I'd find out one day that this is used to treat Lyme disease too—but at this time, it was still years before Lyme would enter my Universe.

IVIG is a human blood product pooled from thousands of healthy donors, scrubbed down to its purest form, and infused into the body through a port that's inserted in the arm and leads directly to the heart. IVIG neutralizes the problematic antibodies in the bloodstream and, therefore, mellows many raging autoimmune diseases. This would, we hoped, prevent my body from attacking my nerves. There were miracle stories on the Internet about how it helped people to walk again, eased their pain, and returned them to a normal life.

A week later I had the surgery to insert the port required to deliver the treatment. A week after that, I started.

For three months, five days a week and eight hours a day, I sat attached to an IV pole in Dr. Ourm's office, hooked up to what Jay and I called the "maybe-miracle." Jay was in between jobs at the time, so I was lucky to have him as my loyal infusion companion. He packed us a bag full of things to help pass the time: playing cards, snacks, my beloved *Golden Girls* DVDs, and a laptop loaded with movies. At lunchtime, he would often visit three different restaurants to pick up my favorites from each.

It was after each infusion that I would find myself curled up into a fetal position, my body seizing with pain, fever, and agony. Dr. Ourm was always as happy about that reaction as Dr. Ashish is with my reaction now, because this was an indication that the treatment was working. My immune system was kicking into high gear and my nerves were being repaired.

You probably already guessed that the IVIG treatment didn't turn out to be the cure. But it did do something, at least. I no longer kicked involuntarily due to muscle spasms and even occasionally had the strength to kick on purpose. Sometimes I was only a seven or an eight on the pain chart. But I was simultaneously going downhill. I developed labored breathing, severely low blood counts, and worsening overall fatigue; impossible to tell whether these were side effects of the IVIG, or of the steroids they gave to control the side effects, or were a brand-new issue of concern. Dr. Ourm sadly admitted defeat and stopped the treatment.

Luckily, the stem cell–induced reaction that has me coiled up into full fetal pose turns out to be much more temporary than in my IVIG days, when every symptom became a new long-standing issue. By the morning after my mega stem cell dose, I am back to my "normal" self, and ready for our New Year's Eve celebration just a few days later. Thank Ganesha!

Because my good Jewish parents can't bear the thought of anyone being alone in their room eating hospital food on a holiday, we have planned a New Year's Eve group dinner in the lobby for all the patients.

Despite the angry thunderstorms that are rattling and lighting up the skies, they insist on venturing out into the flooded city to pick up food for all of us from the Big Chill restaurant—the most American eatery we've found in Delhi. It's located in upscale Khan Market, a thirty-minute tuk-tuk ride from the hospital. Their menu includes everything we miss from home: pizza, pasta, salads, and a tuna melt that I have started to live for. As much as I'm warming to Indian food (so much so that I'm gaining weight from it), it's still no buttery, cheesy, pressed gooey sandwich from the Big Chill.

Mom and Dad are gone for almost two hours while the rest of us sit in the lobby trying not to starve, or to worry that they've been swallowed by the storm. When they finally make it back to the hospital, they are buried in the tuk-tuk, bags of food looped around every shoulder, elbow, and wrist. I run out, covering my head with the hood on my sweatshirt, and help them bring in the goods. They are soaked all the way through as if they have willingly offered themselves up to the hungry monsoon. Apparently it was an arduous tuk-tuk ride through holiday traffic and puddles of rain higher than the tires. Any adventure out into the city is enough in the light of day, let alone on a dark, stormy, busy night.

When the driver realizes they are delivering food to a hospital full of patients, he won't take money for the ride.

During the holidays, it seems that the space between humans is less and we're all more the same than different. Tonight is all about the goodness that exists, no matter who you are or where you're from.

My dad tips him twice as much as the ride itself cost for his kind gesture, and we all wave good-bye as he floats back out into the street. I have always known I have the coolest, most generous and selfless parents in the world. But in this moment, drenched and still fully smiling, they are really showing it off.

We dig into the spaghetti Bolognese (with real marinara sauce and no corn!), fusilli chicken, rich, buttery garlic bread, and tangy Caesar salad. It is nothing less than a foodgasm. We are sixteen virtual strangers, bound by the bond of stem cells and Italian food, sitting around one long table, stuffing carbs into our faces and laughing in awe at the circumstances of our meeting. We are more than friends now, we decide; we are . . . related? I look around the room and wonder what will become of us, not individually, but as a group; as people who might never have chosen each other, save for what has brought us together here. Are these the people you meet who become part of your life forever, as familiar as your siblings and childhood playmates? Or are these the people you match up with only temporarily, when you are all suspended together in the same place, on your way to somewhere else?

The stories circle around the room, all of us getting to know each other more deeply than a passing "hi" in physio or an afternoon tea in the lobby.

A young mother from London proudly reenacts how her two-year-old spoke a complete sentence over the phone that day: "I miss you, Mummy!" She is at the hospital healing from an autoimmune disease that's threatening her life.

A retired police officer from New York is here to restore function in his lower body after an accident left him a paraplegic. He gives us an important tip on how to get out of a speeding ticket: first rule—always admit your mistake; and second rule—always apologize.

It is an early 9 p.m. when we end the night with a toast and New York–style cheesecake. Our New Year's Eve party has been full of joy and laughter, but that doesn't change the fact that we are in a hospital and all have to get up for physio early tomorrow. There is none of the pressure of New Year's Eves past: who to kiss at midnight, or how we'll get home safely after a night of drinking. We're already sober *and* at home—score!

Mom and Dad head back to their bed-and-breakfast and me to my room, but I am wide awake, thanks to the celebrating city and maybe too much sugar from these past few days of party food. I hear fireworks beginning already, but I can only see muted sparks of color through the polluted night sky, and a hint of the brightly lit temple down the street.

I hear the street guru on his megaphone somewhere nearby, hollering his prayer. It echoes through the alleys, around the corners, and back to my room. I soak it up, take it in, and let it reverberate through me. I wonder if it is a special prayer for this special night. He is never out this late. His voice is easily one of my favorite things in this city, a stark contrast to the loud, fast, and erratic noises that siphon out any moments of peace. I feel his slow, steady tone with me long after his prayers fade out of my reach.

As the last few hours of 2007 quickly close in, I realize there isn't going to be a year quite like this one ever again.

It was only nine months earlier that Jay and I were officially over and I was back living with my parents. They had moved from our childhood home up to Northern California among the majestic auburn-colored redwoods and crisp, clean air.

My home might have changed, but the search for my health continued.

Among my recent lab tests, a toxicology report had shown that I had dangerously high levels of benzene in my system. Benzene is a carcinogenic substance that is found in crude oil. How that got into my body is just another mystery on my list of WTFs.

The toxicologist recommended hyperbaric oxygen treatment, which involves breathing pure oxygen in a pressurized environment. Infusing a patient with pure oxygen can help kill infections, clear toxins, and enhance the immune system. It is a well-established treatment for decompression sickness from scuba diving, as well as for serious infections and wounds that won't heal.

I needed twenty sessions at $300 each, and insurance didn't cover it. "We've really got to get this stuff out of you," the toxicologist stressed, as he wiped tears from my cheeks.

Two weeks later and 229 miles from my new home, I found myself sitting with the director of the hyperbaric clinic in Chico, California, seeking another treatment and chasing another cure. Mitch was in his sixties, well dressed, never without a bow tie, and the caring heart behind this treatment center.

I found a place to live nearby, an apartment stuck in the seventies, with shag carpet and dreary cream-colored paint. The cost of the apartment and the treatment swallowed up all my monthly state disability allowance and, as usual, a lot of Mom and Dad's bank account too. This new life was far from the airy three-bedroom house I'd shared with Jay, and even more deflating than being an adult living with my parents.

Every day I drove to the treatment center and climbed into a large metal pressurized oxygen tank with five other patients, each of us wearing a clear hood as if we were part of a hazmat team in a sci-fi movie. Large tubes extended from these hoods and connected us to the tank. For two hours each day, our bodies drank in 100 percent pure O_2.

At first, I felt nothing terribly abnormal for me, only mildly dizzy and majorly nauseated. But it was during the third treatment that things changed. On the third day, I went into the tank feeling my normal version of crappy and came out almost unable to move even a single joint. Every part of my body was inflamed, pulsating, and excruciatingly tender to the touch. I had developed full-blown arthritis in all my major joints. I went from twenty-seven to eighty-seven years old in the two hours I was inside.

I hobbled back to the car and then into my dingy apartment, assuming this was just another crazy reaction from another crazy treatment. I had become desensitized to my body's expressions of discontent. Not only did nothing worry me anymore, but nothing made me pay attention anymore either. I saw my body as uncooperative and unruly, never on my team. I planted myself on my rented couch and didn't move all night.

"Amy, I think you have Lyme disease," Mitch said the next day, sitting at his desk across from me, his chin wrinkled and his face somber.

But, you see, I didn't have Lyme disease. I had seen dozens of specialists at the top institutions in the country. I had even been tested for it years before. Mitch had to be wrong.

"I was tested for it and it came back negative," I told

Mitch, opening my three-inch binder full of medical records and pointing to the results from two years earlier as proof. I carted that medical binder around to every appointment, proud that I had systematically ruled out having every disease on earth and could confirm it for any doctor who offered a new theory. I was always ready to show how far I had gone to find the truth. I pulled open the middle ring, freeing the paper that proved my point, and passed it to him over the desk.

"You got the test done at the wrong kind of lab. Testing for Lyme disease is only accurate when you get it done at a lab that specializes in tick-borne illnesses," Mitch explained, passing it right back to me. "The response you're having to the oxygen treatment seems like a Herxheimer reaction. This happens when a treatment kills the bacterium that causes Lyme disease, and it begins to die off rapidly in your body."

Mitch had become an accidental expert on Lyme disease because, tragically, his son had passed away from it when he was in his twenties. But I couldn't process any of what he was saying. *I am here for benzene toxicity treatment. How can I now have an entirely new disease? And if I have it, am I going to die like Mitch's son? I do not have Lyme, I do not have Lyme*, I repeated in my head.

Yet the more I learned about Lyme, the more it sounded like me.

Borrelia burgdorferi, the bacterium that causes Lyme disease, often burrows deep within the body and can affect all the organs, glands, and systems. It not only attacks and alters the function of the immune system but also evades the very antibiotics that try to kill it. The symptoms mimic hundreds of other illnesses, which makes Lyme disease difficult to diagnose. In fact, Mitch told me that most general practitioners aren't properly educated on it, so the signs and symptoms are often overlooked.

Many specialists on the front lines of treating Lyme believe that, if not diagnosed and treated early, it can trigger other diseases—multiple sclerosis, Lou Gehrig's disease (ALS), and Parkinson's disease. To complicate matters even more, Lyme disease is entrenched in a political firestorm, with doctors disagreeing on testing methods and treatment protocols, and insurance companies refusing to pay for much of the necessary treatment. There is no sure way to treat it; everything is experimental and everyone is shooting in the dark.

I do not have Lyme, I do not have Lyme, I continued, but now more as a prayer than anything else. Because something about me having Lyme disease rang perfectly and absolutely true. I felt it where I feel all the deepest, truest things—in my bones.

It was six weeks later, after more testing, this time from the "right" lab, that I got the truth from Dr. Harr, who was something of a cross between a surfer dude and a scientist, and one of the best Lyme disease specialists in the country.

"You have Lyme disease," Dr. Harr said casually, as if he didn't need a test to tell him. Mitch was right.

Finally, seven years after my very first symptoms, the ones that my doctor said were "maybe hormones" and "probably nothing," I had arrived here. In between then and now had been tens of thousands of dollars in medical bills, endless specialists, broken relationships, failed treatments, and false hopes. But I was finally being diagnosed with what I intuitively knew was *it*. Some wise place within me knew this would be my very last diagnosis.

Lyme disease accounted for every mystery and symptom I'd been chasing for almost a decade. This is the jackpot moment in a chronically ill person's life. It is when you finally find a disease that rolls off your tongue without a shred of doubt. It is the disease that you decide to marry and be loyal to after all the ones that came and went like the wind.

This diagnosis would turn out to give me all the answers I had been seeking, but also none of them at all. Because finally getting the right diagnosis was monumental, but the task of treating the disease at this late stage was even bigger. It was climbing Mount Everest, except your hiking boots are flip-flops and your flip-flops are broken.

I suddenly felt the urge to reach back into my past and

take any of my old diagnoses back. I bargained with the Universe, but there was no swapping allowed.

On top of the nauseating oxygen sessions, which Dr. Harr suggested I continue, he added new treatments: heavy-duty antibiotics and dozens of supplements—pills, tinctures, and powders—all of which seemed to exacerbate my symptoms. Each day became a new kind of nightmare.

I couldn't keep up with the pain, fatigue, detox regimens, side effects, restrictions on what felt like almost every kind of food or drink, and medication schedules (take *this* but not within two hours of *that*; take *this* right before bed on a full stomach; and take *that* three times a day along *with* this, but never in the same three hours as *this*). I had reminders and spreadsheets for what to do, and when—my day full of activities, not one of them pleasurable.

Once I was entrenched in the wild and complex world of Lyme disease, it *became* me—my research project, my wound, my identity. My life started to spin around this disease. Mostly because I was scared that if I took my eyes off it, it might kill me.

I backslid worse than ever before, emotionally and physically. I was devastated that this new diagnosis, which should have been the end of my hardships, was only the beginning. I wanted to run away, but I couldn't even get off the couch. My parents moved into the Chico apartment's second bedroom, taking turns helping take care of me. I painfully straddled the line between desiring my independence and being a child who could not live without her mommy and daddy.

Mom helped lift me in and out of baths full of vinegar and baking soda, trying to leach out the toxic medications and bacteria die-off from my system. The pressure of the mattress in my bedroom was too harsh for my joints, so we propped up my knees, ankles, elbows, and shoulders with pillows on the couch. She slept there with me each night while, as always, my trusty *Golden Girls* DVDs looped on replay. "We're watching this again?" my mom would ask, even though she knew the answer. She waited anxiously outside the bathroom door when I couldn't stop throwing up. She ran out to pick up fettuccini Alfredo, sometimes the only food I wanted, even though I could almost never keep it down.

Dad provided the therapy, jokes, and questionable entertainment, often reading to me from his favorite magazines—*Costco Connection* and *Consumer Reports*. I was sick as hell and didn't know how to help myself, but I did know all about the hottest new TVs and most fuel-efficient cars on the market.

He and I were sitting on either end of the couch one evening watching *Frankie and Johnny* when he looked over at me with a proposition and thoughtful eyes. "Wanna try some weed to see if it helps you feel better?" he asked. My dad's empathy poured out at all times, but most honestly in times of desperation. He usually pulls out the old records and old stories, but that night, it was an old pastime: pot.

He had his medical marijuana license, which all the cool dads have. It afforded him access to the ultrapremium, extra-stinky, grade-A bud.

When I was in high school, a few of my friends and I played hooky from school to get high. When my parents were gone for the day, we hurried into the garage and "borrowed" my dad's prize memento from Woodstock: his ceramic bong, hand-painted with delicate flowers. I carefully carried it onto the back patio, and we all arranged ourselves in a kumbaya circle. Four mind-blowing hits later, I agonizingly watched in slow motion as the bong slipped from my friend's hands and hit the floor, smashing into a messy pile of broken pieces.

He never found out, or he never said anything. Either way, I secretly owed him.

"Okay, I'll try it," I agreed.

My dad rolled a doobie, and I still don't know which was glowing brighter, the joint or his face. His pride over our new father-daughter bonding experience was epic. I took three deep tokes, sucked all the THC I could into my lungs, and waited.

But it didn't relieve the pain. Two hours later, Dad was snoring on the couch, having the deepest sleep of his life, and I was wide awake and bug-eyed, watching the divots in the ceiling come alive.

It was after nearly a year of oxygen treatments and a rigorous Lyme disease treatment protocol that it became clear that I wasn't getting significantly better. I did experience some improvement in cognitive function—the ability to speak and think more clearly—but the rest of me didn't seem to be following.

I spent most of each day using all my might to stay alive. I studied the blossoms on a bubble-gum-pink cherry tree outside my apartment window, wondering if I'd still be there the next day to see it. Sometimes I wished that I wouldn't be. The treatments had likely done all they could do—the antibiotics killing the bacteria, the supplements helping support my organs and glands, and the oxygen detoxing me and bolstering my immune system. But it was not enough. What would repair the damage done to my body? What would turn me, an arthritic, exhausted mess, into the normal healthy person that I deserved to be?

The answer, at this point, was unknown.

That's when we decided to slow all the treatment down to the bare minimum needed to at least try to keep any remaining bacteria at bay. I finished my ninety-ninth hyperbaric oxygen treatment and cut back to only the prescriptions and supplements that were essential.

Within weeks, I stopped vomiting. I could move around by myself with enough painkillers, antinausea meds, and sheer will. I never attained any version of the state of health that I imagined for myself; but without the same level of pain, fatigue, and at least a dozen intense symptoms burdening me, I had spurts of being more functional, waves of feeling slightly less horrible. It felt sometimes like I was living.

From this turning point until I set off for India would be a slow and steady march, coming out of a dark hole and into the tiniest light of day.

Even though I was now free to move away from Chico, I did something that felt surprisingly right: I stayed. I stayed because when I listened closely to my body, Chico felt like home. I stayed because the trees and the long grass called to me. I stayed because I had no reason to leave. And I stayed because something told me that this could be my chance to begin again.

I moved out of my apartment with the lackluster walls and shag carpet, and into a new, light-filled place with a sliding door that opened to a field that showcased the setting sun each evening. I spent time on my patio sipping lemon water, counted stones around my toes at the local creek, and strolled through the farmer's market in Chico's charming downtown. I bought bunches of sunflowers the color of canaries and blackberries so plump that they popped in my mouth when I ate them.

Each blistering summer afternoon, I let the 110-degree heat soak into my aching body and melt the pain into something less intense. I splashed around in the cool water of the pool at my apartment complex. I met Ajay, who would later introduce me to the world of Indian food. I had a friend, Sara, who walked slowly with me through the park. Matt, Chico's favorite massage therapist, worked magic on my resistant muscles. Jeff, who moved here from my childhood neighborhood five hundred miles away, invited me over for barbecues with his friends and taught me how to make the best guacamole on earth. Once I went to a Colbie Caillat concert alone and attempted to dance like the cool teenage girls sitting next to me in tube tops. It wasn't always easy being on my own, but the effort of independence was necessary, something I so desperately needed, even if I didn't always do it well.

How things have changed in just a single orbit around the sun—the year of 2007. Watching the late-night smog dance over Delhi, I trace 2007 backward in my mind: starting with the call when Dr. Shroff said "Come to India now," then to the enchanted island of Maui before that where I serendipitously met Amanda the Stem Cell Messenger, and even earlier than that to my beloved town of Chico when I finally received the Lyme disease diagnosis, and despite it, a little piece of spirit back.

How many individual moments created the tiny waves of motion that would turn the tides of my life? How many times in one year did my destiny quietly change its course, its direction? How many moments of this past year had to be orchestrated perfectly in order to get me to where I am right now? This is the work of the Universe: each junction a perfect culmination of mishaps and synchronicities.

Tonight I am reminded that years go by slowly, and they also move in invisible flashes without any foresight of what is to come. From my hospital room in India, an unknown future is awaiting my arrival.

When the clock finally strikes midnight, the city sets itself ablaze: the sky explodes into a rainbow light show, people rejoice, and dogs howl. From my prime spot at the window, I usher in 2008 with a warm welcome.

Tonight there is joy, and uncertainty, yes; but there is also this indisputable fact: No matter where one is in the world, no matter what has been or what might come next . . . as long as we are alive, there will always remain the purest, most simple opportunity—to begin and begin again.

6

This Brain Is on Fire

It's green! Everywhere I look is green. Lush trees. Vibrant flourishing bushes. And a large reservoir with green . . . murky water. But still, it's green!

We are in Hauz Khas, a large neighborhood a little over a mile from the hospital, but a whole new world. This area can be traced back to the thirteenth century and is scattered with ruins of medieval architecture. At the heart of its centerpiece is a lake. Around the lake are scattered domed tombs of Muslim royalty. Ducks and geese from the reservoir mingle with the tourists who flock here. A group of elementary school–age kids are playing a spirited game of cricket as passersby cheer.

It is on a pleasant Sunday afternoon, under the warm sun, that I and a group of patients have made our way to this hidden sanctuary in the dusty Delhi metropolis, some of us by foot and some by wheelchair. I have no idea how this destination has been under my radar all of this time, but it is the best surprise of my trip thus far. I am in paradise.

I am not a girl who loves roughing it, but I am definitely a girl who loves nature. I grew up by the teal-green ocean in the palm-tree-studded Southern California town of Ventura. Our four-bedroom farm-style house in a middle-class neighborhood was packed with pets of every kind, books, music, and love, perfectly planted among the vibrant orange orchards that became our extended backyard. It was full of mazes that David, Lauren, and I got lost in as kids—and then later as teenagers, where we snuck out to smoke cloves and drink with our friends. As a family, we spent weekends in the nearby Shangri-la town of Ojai, where I was born, surrounded by eight different kinds of emerald-green oak trees. Green is my favorite color and my favorite feeling.

Making our way from the hospital to this glorious mecca, we draw endless stares from locals, and especially children. I am getting accustomed to this, hardly flinching when we weave in and out of dense, pushy crowds, and meet the eyes of people who seem shocked at our presence. Our fair skin is one anomaly in this city, but wheelchairs are virtually a sight unseen. Because of the extreme poverty in India, most disabled people can't afford a wheelchair, which here costs approximately seventy-five American dollars. Our group has six sets of wheels, and it has not gone unnoticed. If my dad were here with us, I'm pretty sure he'd be offering demonstrations of how wheelchairs work. He loves to engage everyone he can find in every kind of conversation. But he's not here, because he is stuck in bed a few blocks away at the bed-and-breakfast, in one of his mysterious depressive episodes. It seems that whatever has been stalking him for the past two decades crosses international borders with ease. As usual, there is no identifiable trigger that caused it, no sign as to when it'll pass. But it will. Mom is holed up with him until it does.

We first arrive at Hauz Khas village, which is at the entrance of this neighborhood and lined with upscale jewelry shops and art galleries. The narrow streets are the color of sandstone and rust.

It is only once you've made your way through the village that endless acres of parkland suddenly open up before you. This part of Hauz Khas covers two levels with expansive green vegetation and terra-cotta-colored, dome-shaped buildings.

On the first level, we see various tombs of minor Muslim royalty from the fourteenth to the sixteenth centuries.

Below that, down several uneven flights of stairs made from brick, sits the murky green lake, originally built as a reservoir to supply water to the local community. Hauz Khas itself was named after this body of water, and the name translates to Royal Lake. The towering trees instantly transport me to the deep forests of Northern California in Mendocino, where there is abundant fresh air and silence. It reminds me of the few months I spent there living with my parents after Jay and I fell apart, trying to heal my tired body and a broken heart. Each day I would walk for hours, ever so slowly, through the woods, trying to see meaning in my new life of incomplete change. It was there among the green canopies, when I felt stripped of everything I knew, that I saw actually quite a lot existed. I found contentment in the little things, like the lizard crossing a fallen log, the tree stump someone had painted pink, and the woodpecker insistent on his work. Sometimes, when you have less, you're able to see more. There had been times in my past, when things were going effortlessly well, that I felt like I should have appreciated what I had more—paused just to feel thankful and maybe even spoke my gratitude out loud. But you can only take it in when you can take it in. And in that very difficult time after Jay and I split up, I was surprised by what I was able to appreciate quite easily. The gaping holes of what I had lost only helped to illuminate the beauty that was still all around.

The scattering of buildings that dot the property

are an explorer's dream—steep steps and sharp corners that reveal stone and brick hideaways—but none of my wheelchair-bound friends can access them. Even the flat areas of dirt are uneven with jagged rocks sticking out of the ground, a danger to vulnerable wheelchair tires. Those of us on foot enjoy being tourists and explore, while the patients in wheelchairs marvel at the view and wave to us from the top tier.

Our afternoon trip is long and feels arduous on my muscles that otherwise only get a workout in physio, but it is worth the delights of greenery in a city seemingly made of dust. It surprises me that on our journey home, I am able to push the wheelchair of a patient to give his caregiver some relief. It feels good to exert myself. My body responds with added strength instead of collapsing under the pressure. But this is not only good for my muscles; it's good for so much more. This world I am living in is beginning to feel like *life*. Today I am just a girl, out with my friends, leaning into the pull of the city. *My* city.

It is this excursion that sets the tone of the first week in the New Year, which unfolds like a leisurely, enjoyable meal. Everything feels simple, slow, and uncomplicated.

That is how I should know things are about to take a turn. Because in India, whether it's times of bliss or times of battle, nothing remains stagnant.

When I see Dr. Shroff the next day in physio, she approaches me with a proposal: "I think we should send you for a brain scan to see what is happening. Your balance is getting better, so it is possible that the oxygen flow is improving! It would be wonderful to take a look and have proof of the efforts."

Since my last scan almost a year ago, I have completed months of heavy-duty antibiotics and hyperbaric oxygen therapy sessions, which should have helped address this exact problem. And now I've had the added benefit of stem cells! I immediately agree to the test, because who doesn't want to see pictures of their healing brain?

The scan turns out to be a four-hour extravaganza, which, if not for my dear mother, would have sent me to the mental ward.

Outside the facility, a two-man floor-washing crew greets us. This is a constant sight in India: men who are washing and sweeping. It happens in buildings and on sidewalks—I've even seen people determinedly sweeping the dusty streets. Nothing ever gets clean here, but it is definitely not for lack of people trying to make it so. Every building has designated staff washing the floors nonstop. An area will be washed and rewashed over and over for the entire day. Sweep, mop, scrub, rinse, then repeat. It happens at the most inopportune times in the most random places.

These two men outside the clinic are painstakingly scrubbing the steps that lead down to the entrance. These steps are a danger already, as the handrail is only a few feet tall, far too low to rest a hand on for support. The stairs are slick with soap and water, adding insult to possible injury. I guess they don't have slip-and-fall lawsuits here. "Take a picture, babe!" Mom screams. She hunches over, reaching for the handrail, which is down by her knees, and ducks into the frame of the camera with a funny face. What I have always loved most about my mom is her ability to see the humor in every situation.

When I was ten, we went on our annual trip to New Jersey to visit all our extended family. My parents surprised us with a side trip to the Amish country in Pennsylvania, where we stayed on a working farm. One afternoon, David and I herded the roaming goats from the field, quietly coaxed them toward our building, and stifled our laughter as we lured them into our room. But they didn't just walk in; they RAN, jumping on the bed and over the furniture, spraying pellets of poop *everywhere*. When Mom saw the commotion, she didn't yell or put us in time-out. Instead, she buckled in hysterical laughter, tears rolling down her face, motioning for my dad to break out the video camera. When we were kids, she used to tell us, "The family that laughs together stays together!" Dad would then interrupt to say, "No, no, the family that farts together stays together!" And we'd all giggle, arguing back and forth about it.

We manage our way down the steps to the scanning facility, planting our feet carefully on each one, and enter the building to hurdle our next obstacle: another bucket of water and another worker, this time bathing the tiles in cough-inducing pine-scented cleaner.

At the front desk, I check in for my appointment, pay my fee, and wait while the receptionist stares at me with no further direction. In this country, to be stared at means one of a few things: *hi*, *sit down*, *I don't know what to say*, or *go away*. If you don't get a stare here, you will likely get the infamous Indian headshake, or head bobble, a repetitive side-to-side tilting of the head. The head bobble is the nonverbal version of Chavi's "fine," meaning *it's all good*, *okay*, *I understand*, and *yes*. I'm finally getting a handle on the subtle idiosyncrasies of the culture here.

I walk away, sitting down with Mom in the waiting area. Eventually a man comes out from the back and calls my name. I follow him on a zigzag path, around yet more mopping, and into a dark, cramped office where a doctor sits in a swivel chair. He doesn't offer me a seat.

"Soooo?" he asks as he spins himself around, hands folded on his stomach, then waits for me to talk.

"I'm here for a SPECT scan. I had one last April in California and need another one to see if anything has changed," I explain.

"Yessss, I know," he confirms. "Dr. Shroff has given me the details. Now, where are your last SPECT results?"

When I explain I don't have them, he lowers his eyes in grave disappointment and says "Ohhhh, that would have beeeeen niiiice" several times in a row. I stand there awkwardly smiling, while he makes his point.

"Yesssss, that would have beeeeen verrrrry niiiice. Verrrrry niiiice." He shakes his head, dragging out each and every word, testing my already short patience.

"I'm sorry. Can I e-mail the records when I get back to the hospital?" I offer, trying to fix it.

"Okaaaaay," he agrees, content with this compromise. "Now we will begin!"

Thank goodness. I'm ready to get on with this and outta here. But then he explains that we will begin with a lot of waiting. First, I have to wait forty-five minutes while they "boil" the dye solution. I immediately wish I didn't know they are going to boil whatever goes into me. I want to ask the doctor why they didn't prepare the dye before I got here, because *that would have beeeeen niiiice*; but I cannot hear it one more time, not even from my own mouth. Next, a technician will inject the dye into my veins, which will take another forty-five minutes to work. This is the "tracer" that will go to my brain and will show up on the images of the scan. Then they will finally perform the scan—which takes another forty-five minutes.

I am starting to worry about all these forty-five-minute time blocks, because in India time is just a suggestion, everything is more relaxed, and things happen when they happen. Dr. Ashish tells the joke that IST (Indian Standard Time) actually stands for Indian Stretchable Time. He is not wrong.

Back in the waiting room, Mom and I sit and watch the floor-mopping crew circle around and around. When they get to our section, they slowly approach us and then push the mops up against our feet as a cue to pop our legs up and allow them to wash underneath. We oblige. When this happens a second time, we smile and do our duty. But by the third time, we are paralyzed with hysterical laughter, and completely unable to cooperate.

Finally, when it's my turn, I am led down a hallway to a small alcove, where the tech administers my injection and directs me to lie still with my eyes closed for forty-five minutes. "No movement, ma'am. You must be very relaxed for accurate test," he tells me.

On his way out, he closes a tissue-paper-thin curtain that is expected to shield me from the commotion of the rest of the facility.

For the next three-quarters of an hour, Hindi music blares in the background and the workers proceed to make more noise than I thought possible. They sing as they shuffle through the hallway area near me to get supplies, flipping the lights on and off repeatedly while yelling something in Hindi to the front desk. I imagine that they're confirming, "Yep, light still works."

There isn't a minute of relaxation that occurs. It's impossible.

When it's time for the actual scan, I'm escorted into a room where the doctor I met earlier is waiting.

"Please remove your jewelry, jacket, and shoes," he says in a curt tone, pointing to the table. I feel immediate relief. During my first week in India, I got an MRI with a technician who pointed to a sign next to my dressing room: PLEASE REMOVE ALL YOUR UNDERGARMENTS. What?! I'd never had to remove my bra and underwear for MRIs at home. This didn't seem legit at all, but what could I do? I stared at my pink-and-teal-striped underwear, debating. With the door bolted shut, I followed the directions, the whole time hearing my mother's voice shrieking in my head: "What, just because a man tells you nicely to take off your underwear, you do it?"

I lie down on the table. Back home, the directions for this test are simple: keep your head as straight as you can, and try to lie still. But here the technician trusts me with nothing. He straps my head into a cagelike contraption, tightening Velcro strips over my forehead and chin. He stuffs cotton beside each of my ears to keep me from moving. I don't consider myself claustrophobic, but in this moment, I am. A radio station is full of static in the background, the printer is jamming, and the fluorescent lights are glaring through my eyelids. No one notices any of it. "Don't move for the next forty-five minutes," they tell me. "Stay frozen. It's very necessary."

The test is physically painless, but mentally exhausting. I can't move my head in this cage, my jaw hurts from clenching, and there is a giant piece of machinery hovering so close to my face that it's skimming the tip of my nose.

Eventually I am done and they set me free. "When you send me your last results, I will provide the new ones," the doctor says. My mom and I leg it out of there as fast as we can.

It is later that evening, after I've e-mailed my part of the bargain, that he replies:

Ms. Amy, I have attached your updated report!

I am excited! Mostly to see proof of my progress, but also to have results this fast. At home, they are always sent directly to the doctor, who then discusses them with the patient. Patients never get this kind of service: e-mailed reports—on the same day—directly from the facility!

I'm about to see why.

My brain has gotten worse since last April, not better.

Last time, I had only a single area of reduced blood flow and oxygen to my brain. Now I have three.

My lungs choke. Heat rushes to my head. My brain is on fire with panic.

I have a severe case of scanxiety. *Scanxiety*: noun: *an undesirable emotional or physical reaction to scan results*. I am pacing in my room, reading and rereading the document, while erratic sobs leak out of me. I call my mom, leave a message for Dr. Shroff, and fax Dr. Harr back home. Then I disappear right back into my fear sphere, a place where I have absolutely zero inability to be calm, rational, or reasonable. This is where I go when it feels like there's nowhere else to run. My worries, doubts, and most ominous questions wait for me there, tantalizing me with addictive worst-case scenarios and outcomes. For some reason, despite all efforts to avoid it, this crazy mental space is a familiar home that pulls me in.

I start asking questions that I have no hope of answering alone.

What does this mean?

Why are things worse?

How could this be?

Who is to blame?

Will this ever end?

"It's not *that* bad," Dr. Shroff tries to convince me the next day when she comes to my room. But what I hear is, "It's *that* bad."

Her consolation fixes nothing. My brain is still on fire.

Dr. Shroff reassures me. "The stem cells will start to help replenish blood flow to your brain and revive the tissue so it can absorb more oxygen. Just try to be patient."

It is a few hours later that I receive a fax back from Dr. Harr's office.

The note says:

Amy—

Different facilities perform and interpret the scans in different ways. You're not comparing apples to apples. Use this scan as your baseline and get another scan before you go. Stop worrying.

Dr. Harr

I should feel comforted, but I don't. I am angry with my body and the doctors. *It's easy for them to say these things,* I think, *because it's not their brain.* When you are twenty-eight years old, you don't want anything wrong with your brain, even if it's "not that bad."

I think back on all the years of love, support, and compassionate words I've received, remembering how hard it is to know what to say to someone who is in pain. Before I got sick, I too spoke some of these questionable consolations to others. And maybe, accidentally, a time or two since. When we don't know how to fix things for another person, we sometimes end up spitting out clichés, not as condemnations but as offerings of love. I'm guilty as charged. "It's not that bad" is a well-meaning sympathy any of us might extend when we're worried that it really *is* that bad. It's not the worst offender I've heard, but it's definitely on the list, and I have quite the list:

"I could never do what you are doing."

Honestly, I'm no superhero. You could totally rock this too, if you had to. In fact, we could all do anything if we absolutely had to. I once thought I could never do what I'm doing either, except for now I don't have a choice and that's exactly how I'm doing it in the first place. Some nights when I go to bed, I think to myself, *I cannot do this, not even for one more day.* Eventually I fall asleep . . . and then . . . I wake up with a life that is just waiting for me to wade through all over again. You do it because even when—especially when—you think you can't, you're somehow still making it happen. And you do it every minute of every day—no breaks allowed—because if you don't, every single thing that you've barely just been holding on to might fall apart too.

"You'll see, one day we'll look back and laugh at this."

We *might* think it is funny one day—but, depending on how this goes, we also might not. So unless we are truly experiencing a serious humor drought, let's not count on laughing just yet. If anyone gets to laugh at this one day, it's gonna be me—but I'll invite you over to help if I need it. For now, though? This is still so not funny.

"It could always be worse—just look at so-and-so."

Sometimes we just need to have a guilt-free pity party for ourselves—tissues, sappy movies, and ice cream in abundance. We need to cry and scream, even if there are other people out there who have it way worse. If you want to be a real friend, just bring over all mint chocolate chip ice cream, please?

"This time in your life was meant to be."

I can *so* get on board with "meant to be." I truly can. But the thing about "meant to be" is that most of us apply that one only when we feel like doing so. And lately, I seriously don't feel like it. I cannot see how physical and emotional torture is meant to be. Not yet, anyway. If I find out that this crisis is really awesome sauce in disguise, I will be super stoked. But for now, the only thing I can believe is meant to be is getting my life back or winning the lottery.

"God doesn't give you more than you can handle."

I love this idea. But if God is even really up there at all, he certainly doesn't feel like a great judge of who can handle what right now—especially if there's any chance God thought it was okay to hand this horror to me in the first place. I respectfully think he might have to sit out for this call.

"Attending church or finding spirituality might help."

I know some people find great solace in religion, and I honor that completely. I've always wanted to be one of them. But in the midst of crisis, I can't do it. So, no. Just no. Also, if I go to church, I might find more people who insist that if only I'd been attending all along, this might not have happened. Plus, I'm Jewish.

"Tomorrow will be better."

This is unlikely, based on my experience yesterday. Being miserable today, it's hard to see how twenty-four hours could change all that much. If tomorrow is better, I'll come back to you and apologize for rolling my eyes; but unless you hear otherwise, assume it turned out the same as the day before. And the day before that.

But here's the thing. There's something funny about this list that I think you should know. Years from now, when I'll be less adamant about what I know and more open to what I don't, I will believe everything on it.

In the meantime, while there are endless wrong things to say, it was my friend Anita who taught me that there is always one *right* thing we can try instead.

It was many years ago, during my IVIG treatment, when she asked with genuine concern, "How are you feeling?" "Horrible," I decided to say truthfully, out of character for me, and with guilt for doing so.

"Well, that fucking sucks," she replied without a filter,

leaving her statement there in the air with a huge space of awkward silence looming behind it. This silence gaped . . . wide . . . open. If this were me, I would have run to its rescue and said something else. *Quick! Fix this space! It needs help! Say more! It's drowning and only I can save it!* Anita just left it alone, teaching me that when someone is in pain, the best and most unexpected consolation is to simply meet them right where they are.

The next afternoon, no matter how hard I try to convince myself that things are "not that bad" or that one day this will be funny, none of it is true. Everything still sucks and my brain is still on fire.

I have just woken up from a nap when I hear a sharp knock on my door.

An older Indian woman makes her way in, flipping on the light as she enters. She has long, thick, silver hair pulled back in a low ponytail, and is carrying a huge silk purse and wearing intricately patterned Indian attire.

"Dr. Shroff has sent me," is the first thing she says, in a raspy voice. Then, "I am Dr. Nittali. I have been a physician for thirty years." She starts pulling the plastic chair from the corner of my room right over to the foot of my bed. She feels closer to a presence than a person—like a spirit, wrapped tightly in a sari.

I sit up in my bed, relieved that Dr. Shroff has sent

another doctor to evaluate me and confirm that we have nothing to be concerned about.

"Don't worry. I know you are going to get well," she states. "It must be hard to feel so sick and look somewhat normal, yes?"

I have no idea why she is here, but as she relaxes into her chair, I can tell that she's crystal clear about it.

"Yes," I answer. I don't think about it often, but what she says strikes me deeply. Doctors have often commented on how "healthy" I look as an addendum to why they are so confused about my dismal blood tests and dysfunctional body. "I'd never be able to tell you were sick if I didn't know your medical history," they'd say. I never leave the house without my hair and makeup perfected and my nails painted. I think a lot of that came from always wanting to look good for Jay, to play the part; but then it became my signature. *Feels like hell, but looks great. Falling apart on the inside, but at least still pretty on the outside.* It was the only thing left I could control.

"I am here to teach you," she says. I am beginning to feel like I am in a made-for-TV movie. I see at this point that she is definitely not here about my brain, or to talk me out of worrying about it.

"Never forget the power of self," Dr. Nittali continues. I am slightly suspicious of Dr. Shroff's motives in sending this mysterious, wise woman. Still, I am sitting cross-legged on my bed, a good, attentive student. Dr. Nittali is disarming, gentle, and receptive.

"Nothing is by chance," she adds, with no further explanation. "Do you know Buddhism?"

"I do," I say, flashing back to my teenage years when I counted mala beads and my favorite books were *Be Here Now* and *The Jew in the Lotus*. I feel its soft comfort, its familiarity, its goodness. I wonder how I drifted so far from that time in my life when I had something of such substance to cling to.

"The essence of Buddhism is the understanding that we all have the ability to transform our suffering. I study Nichiren Buddhism," she explains. "We use *daimoku*, the chanting of specific words to activate joy and freedom even in the face of suffering. This chanting can reveal one's state of inner Buddhahood: enlightenment in your own life. It is freedom. It is already there and always available. Chanting awakens us to it."

I nod and try to take it all in.

"First, I want to share something with you to demonstrate its power," Dr. Nittali says, launching right into a story I'm totally unprepared for.

She starts, "My husband died, twice."

Died twice?

"He was suffering terribly with ALS, a terminal disease," she goes on.

She explains that she tried to fill him up with love and stem cells and everything in between, but he was still declining.

She began to chant vigorously each day. But in the early morning hours of October 13 of last year, Dr. Nittali's husband suffered cardiac arrest and died—then was miraculously revived and put on life support, with little chance of recovery and the likelihood of severe brain damage.

"But my daughter and I were confident in the power of *daimoku*, so we chanted with faith and conviction. We based our practice on a quote from Nichiren's writings: *Life is the most precious of all treasures. Even one day of life is worth more than ten million ryō of gold.* Based on this, we prayed to prolong his life."

They chanted for miracles.

Members and leaders of their community came to the hospital to chant with them. The group chanted in shifts around the clock to keep the energy, and him, alive.

Her eyebrows perk up at the climax of the story.

"Slowly and steadily, he began to come back to life. His faith began to regenerate. He began to chant within his heart," she tells me. "He was released from the hospital on a small portable ventilator with no brain damage whatsoever. He had a glow on his face that was completely out of proportion to someone in intense suffering. A miracle."

He was then transferred to Dr. Shroff's stem cell clinic as an inpatient. And from his room, Dr. Nittali shared their practice of faith and chanting with hospital staff, other patients, their families, and visitors.

This past October, exactly one year after he beat the odds and survived, Dr. Nittali's husband died again.

"It was not until after his second death," she says, "that I understood he could leave only when he was sure that my daughter and I had grown in faith, enough to face the world without him."

Faith. Appearing and reappearing. Over and over. Showing up in different forms, different words, and different offerings. It always comes back.

"Nothing is by chance," she reminds me, finishing a story that has me caught between heartache and joy. "The Universe is shifting to bring you what you need to heal yourself, so then you will be able to move on and do bigger things."

When she says this, I actually feel that somehow, already, she is part of *my* shifting.

There is no space to ask questions or express emotion before she invites me to practice.

"Now we will chant," she says, with a slight intonation

in her voice as if it could be a question. "The words are *Nam myoho renge kyo.*"

I don't know what it means, but I follow her lead. We chant, first slowly and then much faster. I feel the energy shift around me. Our synchronized chanting creates a steady hum in the room, and the presence of something transformational is palpable.

I lose all awareness of time, and when I finally open my eyes, it feels as if I've been somewhere else all along. Suddenly, and without much effort, I feel a sort of peace I've never felt before. I am no longer obsessing about the brain scan. Actually, I am hardly even thinking about anything at all—a rarity for me.

"I suggest you continue every day and stay aware of miracles," she says as she begins to get up.

"Thank you, I will," I promise her.

I don't want to let this guru walk out of my room and my life forever. But I do, because it also feels wrong to clutch on to her when she has just given me what feels like everything she has.

Nam myoho renge kyo translates to "I devote myself to the Lotus Sutra," often referred to as "the king of the sutras." It is a scripture of hope that reminds us we all have an inherent Buddha nature, the ability to access our own deep inner wisdom and live an enlightened life.

I immediately begin to follow Dr. Nittali's advice:

chanting every day as I stay aware of miracles. And then I start to see them.

First, the terrorist rat that has been invading my room is finally caught. Thankfully, it is captured with a humane cage and let free outside—probably to return soon, but I am happy for the momentary success. It has now been proven that people and animals have at least one solid thing in common—they can't resist a good piece of cheese. Finally, a win for the humans! It is with this accomplishment that I am able to move back into my room full-time, and can rest easy.

Second, I have discovered a microwave—on the hospital roof! I can't believe that I've been struggling with food for almost six weeks now, and the answer to my problems has literally been six feet above my head all along. Up one flight of stairs, with no elevator access, and directly above my room, I've discovered a rooftop deck with a view of Green Park. In the far right corner, there is a small afterthought of a room that sits empty, except for a few stacks of dishes and the food-zapping wonder from home. Goodbye, one-dish kettle creations! I can now reheat my Big Chill leftovers and even make popcorn for my evening TV marathons of *Family Ties*, *Friends*, and *Seinfeld*. My inflatable chocolate cake can save me now in two minutes or less if I need it!

And last, but not least, after just two days, the fire in

my brain subsides. My head feels like it has released ten pounds of mental pressure. The uncontrollable angst rushing through me turns off like a water spigot that has run dry. None of it exists anymore.

The erratic ups and downs of the past few weeks have been draining, frustrating, and disheartening. But it is becoming clear that I still need them. I need them because it is only through them that I come out with new perspective, confidence, and hope. I need them because they break me from my desire for control, when I cannot break it for myself. I need them, because without them, I am without the impetus to push myself forward.

Each night, staring at the bright blue wall in my hospital room, I chant myself to sleep.

Nam myoho renge kyo.

I chant because, from day to day, my stillness is still so fragile.

Nam myoho renge kyo.

I chant because somewhere inside me, they say, my enlightened self resides.

Nam myoho renge kyo.

I chant because if there really is a way to transform my own suffering, I want it.

Nam myoho renge kyo.

I chant because I am starting to see that when my brain is on fire, I am the extinguisher.

7

Take It

I am dying. This is the end. My body is giving up or something is killing me. These are the recurring thoughts that I have for almost three days straight during my sixth week in India while I am hanging over the toilet bowl vomiting uncontrollably.

I focus my gaze on my little elephant figurine on the bathroom windowsill, glowing with her brilliant colors and confidence. I need to be reminded of overcoming obstacles pretty much all the time here, but especially right now.

I am shaking, sweating, and so disoriented that I can't see where the door is. Whatever has gotten me is destroying me quickly.

Three sisters are standing over me debating what to do.

"She look sooooo sick," they chatter to each other in

their small, kind voices, with their heads turned away as if I can't hear them. "Should we call doctor now?" They discuss. Then a long pause ensues while they watch me eject my insides. Again and again.

In between rounds of throwing up, and without full coherence, my brain launches into autosearch mode trying to figure out why this is happening. Craziness ensues.

Could it be the malaria-prevention pills I've had to take here?

Is it a side effect of my high-dose IV antibiotics?

A reaction to the stem cells?

Wait! I bet it's yeast overgrowth in my body.

A herx reaction?

Yes, that's probably it.

Or maybe not.

Is my body telling me I need a break?

Or that it needs something else?

Is my body saying anything at all?

I have figure-it-out fatigue. Decoding my body is officially a job I don't want anymore. After years of being unsuccessful, it is clear I'm not very good at it anyway.

I give up.

In times like this, I often run to my parents—not because they'll have any answers, but because they always make me feel better. I realize that now, even when I'm a grown woman, they are still my biggest source of comfort.

But, as planned, they left for home a few days ago, so I am entirely alone in India now. Our last big hurrah was dinner at the splashy Taj Palace Hotel, where we devoured fresh seafood from Mumbai and crisp, chilled white wine. When the day finally came for them to leave, after six weeks of family bonding, insane ups and downs, and incredible excursions, I was surprised at how ready I was. Not because I didn't want them here, but because the roots I've grown in Delhi would help me make it on my own. We kissed good-bye and nobody cried. Because in saying good-bye, there was infinitely less to cry about than six weeks ago when we first said hello to India together.

But now, in this bathroom, I want them back badly. I am weak, scared, and afraid I might never see them again.

"I seeeee. . . ." One of the sisters quickly points at me and then turns to the other two, circling around her eyes with her fingertip. She whispers loudly to them, "She not have any makeup on. Ah!" They all sigh in dramatic relief, realizing that I might not be quite as badly off as I seem. Apparently, my face without makeup is more worrisome and shocking than me vomiting uncontrollably right in front of their eyes.

This is the first time anyone here has seen me without makeup, stripped of mascara and, seemingly, any eyelashes. In fact, this is one of the few times anyone except my family has seen me without makeup. This is what I *actually* look like when I'm not trying to look perfectly held together.

It is not long before Dr. Ashish and Dr. Shroff are both at the doorway.

"This looks like Delhi belly, yes?" Dr. Ashish and Dr. Shroff mumble to each other, with grave concern on their faces. Delhi belly is the dreaded curse caused by eating contaminated food or drinking unfiltered water here. It is beyond my comprehension that anything could be powerful enough to be doing *this* to me. It is also beyond my comprehension that I could have contracted this in the first place.

I've survived almost two months with the alluring smell of street vendor food and didn't cave in and taste a single thing. I peel or boil everything I put in my mouth. I only go to restaurants that serve bottled water on the tables and use filtered water in the kitchen. I brush my teeth with bottled water and pour scorching water from my teapot over the dishes I wash in the shower with tap water. I use antibacterial wipes on my hands (and my fruit) obsessively. And the staff makes all the food I eat here in the hospital.

But if this really is Delhi belly, it should be the world's most sought-after biological weapon. It. Is. Brutal.

The irony of this is that I have finally fallen in love with Indian food! The meals they have been sending from the other hospital are phenomenal. It turns out that Indian food not only satisfies my taste buds, it also helps me feel integrated into this country. I even bought some spices from the market to bring home.

All the Delhi-related enamor that I've built up over the past six weeks instantly disappears with this last gift the city has given me. I am back to asking this very real question: *How many more days can I take in this polluted city so far from the sunshine of California, my own doctors, and the arms of my favorite people?*

Hooked up to an IV of fluids, I sleep sitting up in case I have to run into the bathroom in a hurry. At one point, I'm too weak to make it and get sick into a plastic bag hanging on the end of my bed. My new nose ring plunges in and, after temporarily considering its retrieval, I deem it a lost cause. If I survive this, I will get a shiny new nose ring to celebrate.

It takes a carousel of nurses, doctors, and antivomiting medication before things begin to calm down . . . an entire forty-eight hours after it started. I can finally eat tiny bites of chapati, sip water infused with electrolytes, and not worry that I will be dead soon.

After living with Lyme disease for so long, I have become accustomed to how delicate my body is. Sometimes I am weathered and worn even after a choppy car ride. I cannot imagine recovering from this battering. I predict that my hips will hurt from kneeling on the cold bathroom floor, the Lyme will rear its ugly head because of the stress on my immune system, my ribs and back will feel cracked from overexertion, and my stomach, raw from all the medications I've taken over the years, might never be able to handle an Indian spice again.

When I wake up on day three, fully prepared to be debilitated, I am astonished. I open my eyes, touch my feet to the floor, and walk effortlessly to the bathroom. I stand over the sink and look deep into the mirror, gaze fixed on a face that is the same face of the day before, but also different. I put toothpaste on my toothbrush and pour bottled water over it.

It is with a mouth full of foamy toothpaste that it hits me. I have awoken for the first day in years without any conscious awareness of being sick. When I focus on the feeling, I discover that I am not without physical symptoms—but I have a clear feeling that I am no longer illness itself. What I have on this day is a distinct feeling of health, the one I'm always seeking, the one that's been missing from inside of me for as long as I can remember. *This is it.*

I know what I have to do next.

Still in my pajamas, I throw on my shoes and run downstairs to find Dr. Shroff. Despite all our conflicts and tensions, she is still the first one I want to see. All my bitterness toward her for the nagging lectures has disappeared. It is wherever my nose ring is now. I am not sure exactly why I have this sudden need for her, but all I know in this moment is that I do.

"Dr. Shroff!" I call as I see her in the lobby. I am discombobulated and disheveled. I am also overjoyed. "I think I am better!"

"I do too," she says calmly, smiling, as if she knew it all along. Her cheeks are full and she lights up.

Saying this out loud makes it real. This feeling is what I've been chasing and what I want. But this feeling is also something that I am scared of. Because, what if it doesn't last? And . . . what if it does? This feeling changes everything.

It's the first time I've had this feeling in as long as I can remember, but it's not the first time someone has tried to convince me that I should be feeling it.

It was almost two years ago that Jay and I took a Hail Mary trip to Chicago, where the winds are so powerful they slap your face and you have to lean into them as you walk just to keep your balance. I had officially grown out of treatment options in California.

Northwestern Memorial Hospital is on the Magnificent Mile, an upscale section of the city's infamous Michigan Avenue. The hospital is home to a stem cell transplant program for autoimmune diseases.

During a late-night Internet search, Jay discovered

a blog written by a woman with health issues similar to mine. Her story included a stem cell transplant with Dr. Yu at Northwestern. This type of stem cell transplant, used only under very specific circumstances, requires patients to undergo intense chemotherapy treatment to kill off a dysfunctional immune system in order to build a new and mightier one.

The treatment was hard-core in both commitment and promise—and I was honestly worried that I didn't have the will for it. But Jay never entertained that possibility. In Jay's eyes, there was never anything I couldn't do. Even though I sometimes doubted how happy he was in our relationship, I never doubted that he loved me. He was always trying to find a way for me to live.

It was on the third day at Northwestern, after thorough exams and blood work, when the head of the department, Dr. Yu, broke the news to us.

"Your case is too complex," he said in a thick Japanese accent.

I was a *case*, not a person anymore.

I was too sick to survive the treatment, he explained. "Your body is not strong enough to withstand the chemotherapy. You would need to start off in better shape to make it through," he told me with a drooping face full of regret.

Although I accepted his recommendation as a patient,

I did not accept it as a human being. How could I have to be in "better shape" to be salvageable? If I were in better shape, I wouldn't need a new immune system.

A month later, the phone rang and I picked it up to hear Dr. Yu's voice on the other end. I momentarily thought he was calling to say we should give the treatment a try. Maybe he had changed his mind. But Dr. Yu was calling to tell me he was moving to Japan. We would end up losing touch after this call; but before that, he proposed an idea.

"I think you should go to Mayo Clinic in Minnesota! They will know how to handle you there. There is something that we are missing."

That is how I ended up at the Mayo Clinic two months later, eating radioactive scrambled eggs for breakfast.

The Mayo Clinic in Rochester, Minnesota, is the crème de la crème, the Ritz-Carlton of hospitals. It's as shiny on the inside as it is on the outside. The floors look like they have been polished for days. The clinic, ten million square feet over the entire medical campus, is an entire city for sick people. There are more than thirty thousand medical staff employed. Chandeliers hang from the ceilings. My hopes were pinned higher than the highest key on the baby grand piano in the lobby. I was conquering a whole new state, rotating through a lineup of different specialists over a week's time, so they could work together to figure out the puzzle of my health.

"Bon appétit!" the nurse shrieked, her brunette curls bouncing as she shrugged her shoulders with excitement. Reaching over to my mouth with her gloved hand, she instructed me to open wide. "Ahhhh," she mouthed, showing me how.

This was my first test of the day, a gastric emptying study, to try to identify the cause for the near-constant nausea I'd had on and off for years. The radioactive eggs would light up through my digestive system and be captured through several scans. Yep, the eggs were literally radioactive.

"It's like poison," she said, smiling. "They can't touch your lips or my hands."

Yum! A radioactive blue plate special, I thought as I opened my mouth, closed my eyes, and swallowed.

There were many tests and doctor visits at the Mayo Clinic, but what happened in the neurology department turned out to be a completely unpredictable plot twist. Inconceivable, in fact.

"We start from scratch here. I don't need these!" the lanky neurologist barked at me with a hearty Italian accent. Her short, dark hair quivered in response, right along with me. She slammed my sacred medical binder of records shut and handed it back to me.

Mom was sitting on the stool in the corner, stiff and uncomfortable. Dad was at the nicotine clinic for his on-again, off-again smoking habit; but I wondered if he'd be able to crack the doctor if he was here. He could make anyone soften. We needed him now.

I was convinced that Dr. Downer (full disclosure: this is not her real name) was a robot with a computerized brain, complete with a library of medical knowledge but no emotional backup drive.

I was used to being babied by my doctors. They usually hugged me when I cried. She didn't seem to want to know me, or care if I thought one way or another about her. She cared about diagnostic testing. She cared about what my symptoms were and nothing else.

When she was done with my consultation, she handed me a list of tests I'd never heard of and told me to return the next day when they were complete. "See you tomorrow," she said as she left the room. Still, we got not even a hint of a real live person.

The next day, I returned to a diagnosis I'd never received before. It was the opposite of anything I could have imagined. It remains, to this day, the most unthinkable pronouncement I would ever get.

Diagnosis: normal.

"You are out of shape," Dr. Downer said with no excitement or bewilderment at all. "Severely deconditioned, but otherwise fine," she confirmed.

She started to rattle off proof. "Your blood counts are

normal, your inflammation markers are normal, your urine analysis is normal. Your nerve studies are also normal."

Three months earlier in Chicago, I was too weak to survive a treatment, and now I was normal?

I sat cold and unable to speak. Mom gasped, and I thought I heard an "Oy vey."

I stayed quiet with her pause.

"Your problem has been a combination of things, but now you are fine," Dr. Downer wrapped up.

"So . . ." I started, planning to recap, but couldn't. "I don't understand," I finished, a little bit scared of her reaction.

"Your problems now are due simply to a severely deconditioned body. It is using every ounce of strength just to maintain function. A vicious cycle. Okay?" she said sharply, biting her lip and at the end of her patience. "Pain from the disease caused lack of activity, which caused atrophy, resulting in more pain."

It began to sink in. Dr. Downer was telling me that, despite feeling sick, tired, and miserable, I was . . . disease-free.

"You will make a full recovery," she promised with certainty, slapping her hand on my patient folder to signal that the conversation was over. Case closed.

As she started to stand up from her chair, I finally broke my silence.

"How did you find this but no one else has? Why did the tests keep finding abnormalities if I'm okay? Are you sure?" I asked in succession, my onslaught of questions coming faster than my brain could process them. How could other doctors have found so many problems and she had not?

"Whatever you had is now gone," she repeated, refusing to discuss at any length what anyone else had found. "I am only able to confirm that you are now disease-free."

I began to cry in overwhelm as Dr. Downer watched, her eyebrows furrowed. Her days were usually spent diagnosing some of the world's most terrible illnesses.

I was her lucky day, and she was not going to let me ruin it for her.

"Do you want me to tell you something bad? Would you be happy then?" she questioned with cynicism. "You require a serious pain-rehabilitation program, consisting of major physical therapy. You can start with aquatic therapy, if you must. But we will get you back! Do you want this?!" she yelled like a drill sergeant.

These were the words I heard next, from inside my head: *You are at the Mayo. They are the best. They are the best in the world and the Mayo doesn't lie. THIS IS WHAT YOU WANT. JUST TAKE IT, YA CRAZY. JUST TAKE IT.*

It felt like an hour had passed, but it was only seconds before I answered, "Yes, that is what I want." Mom nodded in eager support. We were all on board.

When I agreed to be cured with no reasonable explanation and to accept her wisdom as my own convenient truth, she seemed to move slightly closer to some version of compassion. Dr. Downer had just one final set of instructions: "There is only one thing you can do now: stop being sick and heal." She said this as if it were so simple and obvious, it made me momentarily question what I had been wasting my time doing all of these years.

I don't have to tell you that, while maybe the Mayo Clinic didn't lie, they definitely didn't know the truth either. No amount of physical therapy or sheer will that followed Dr. Downer's promise would be enough to make my new diagnosis of good health come true.

But on this day in India, when I step out of bed and into the feeling of health, I sense the wisdom of this advice again: *THIS IS WHAT YOU WANT. JUST TAKE IT, YA CRAZY.*

So I do—because this time, no one is *telling* me it's there. This time, I feel it for myself, and it is absolutely, without a doubt, real.

It will be a long time before I look back on Delhi belly and see it as a gift. But when I do, I actually won't see Delhi belly at all. I will instead see those three days of violent illness as my storm before the calm. I will see the vomiting as my body's opportunity to eject years of Lyme disease and all that came with it: the pain, the sorrows, and the broken dreams. Despite much resistance and sometimes refusal, this was my body's way of putting my Whac-A-Mole mallet down and stepping out of the game. From that day forward, the Lyme monsters don't own me anymore.

·   ·   ·

IT IS THE new, more vibrant me who welcomes my sister-in-law, Tatiana, to Delhi. It is a few days after my astonishing renewal.

"Siiiiis!" she squeals when she first sees me, looking straight toward my sparkling new nose stud.

She can't believe how much healthier I seem compared to when she saw me last. I was a wreck. But now I am finally living in a somewhat decent body, weaned off my mind-numbing meds, in less pain, and ready to share normal, healthy-person adventures with her.

When I introduce Tatiana to the other patients and their family members, I refer to her as "my sister." You can almost see their wheels turning. How is this tall and slender Mexico City native, with jet-black hair, a notable accent, and dark skin, related to this short, green-eyed blonde? *Adopted?* I feel people wonder. But the truth is, I've never thought of her as an in-law. When David brought Tatiana home to meet our family three years before, she proved herself a perfect misfit and instant member of our tribe.

Instead of shaking my dad's hand, she yelled "Daddy!" and embraced him as if they were being reunited after years apart. We have been *sisters* ever since.

It takes Tatiana only two days to adjust to the time change, the city, and the food. She is an avid traveler and practiced at surviving with only a backpack and a map. This is nothing for her. *This* is where it's obvious that we are not blood relatives.

We make big plans and start right away. First we hit the zoo, where I get the biggest compliment I've gotten in a long time. "Shakira! Helloooo, Shakira!" several young schoolboys holler in our direction. When I finally realize it's me who has been incorrectly identified as the epic musical sensation, I, completely flattered, kindly deny any relation. No one is buying it. We spend the rest of our visit heading toward the exit, trying to outrun my new fan club. Next we visit the three-story mall, eyeing the latest in Indian fashions and sucking down traditional vanilla lattes from Starbucks. And then we do what should be done for all sisterly reunions: book appointments for a relaxing spa day.

We arrive at the ayurvedic center outside of town via a taxi, through a cloud of smoke, dozens of bicycles, a cow stopping three cars, a trash windstorm that temporarily blocks our view, and a driver who has no idea where he is going. He has basically taken us for an hour-long joy ride—something that happens to me often here.

Finally pulling up to an authentic-looking wooden cottage, we are ready for the most rejuvenating experience to be had in all of Delhi. We check in at the front desk and are soon following our massage therapists into rooms across the hall from each other. "Enjoy, sis!" I shout to her as her door closes.

Ayurveda is an ancient Indian system of health care that includes healthy living along with therapeutic measures that relate to physical, mental, social, and spiritual harmony. This is exactly what I need right now.

It is only minutes into my spa experience that I have a realization: all massages are definitely not created equal. Imagine cushy padded massage tables, gentle manipulation of sore muscles, soft towels draped over your body, relaxing music, and total peace.

Now erase every speck of that image from your mind.

Ayurvedic spa–reality is lying on a cold, rock-hard, wooden table not quite wide enough for your entire body, naked except for the tiny paper underwear that has been provided, with two women—one on each side of you— rapidly speaking Hindi, their hands strong enough to break bones, pummeling your flesh into mush. There are no sounds of waterfalls. There is no hunky masseuse. There is only the echo of your own thighs violently and repeatedly slapping together.

I later find out that the uncomfortable table, called a

droni, is necessary because of the amount of massage oil that's used, which by the way only enhances the echoes of jiggling thighs. The women rhythmically knead each muscle of my body. They are sparing no oil or pressure around areas so delicate that I'd normally want them covered up. Instead, they massage confidently, as if they own every inch of my vulnerable body. They are chatting in Hindi, I'm guessing about whether I knew what I was getting into.

In the past, I would have been more self-conscious about something like this, but some of my modesty has faded. Now I look at my body and I think, *I cannot believe it has survived so much.* This perspective is a beautiful thing. I wish I had found it earlier than now.

Next comes a treatment ritual called *shirodhara*, in which lukewarm herb-infused oil is poured over the forehead. It's done in a continuous stream using a special rhythmic swaying movement that's beyond bliss. During this, I relax into a nearly comatose state and forget that I am naked and doused in oil—in front of strangers. The oil is liquid silk being cascaded over my head, and if it never ended, it would be too soon. By the time it is over, I have forgotten the discomfort of the first part of my treatment and am ready to do it all over again.

When my time is up, I attempt to gracefully step down from the table, but instead I end up clumsily sliding off.

My massage therapists give me a small towel to wrap myself in and point me across the hall toward a sauna. It resembles a time machine from an old sci-fi movie. I awkwardly maneuver my way into the steamy box while the ladies spin me out of my towel and stand at attention next to me. After ten minutes of profuse sweating, they signal for me to come out. I take a cold shower with the powdered soap they provide—as they watch. I wish I knew any kind of Hindi term for "Please avert your eyes for just a minute!"

When I am done, they reunite me with Tatiana. I feel like I haven't seen her in days. Her expression is unfamiliar to me, even after all the years we've known each other.

"Hi," I say hesitantly, trying to read how she is feeling. I get no response, her big brown doll eyes only glancing in my direction. I try to make her smile by silently laughing and rolling my eyes toward the hallway with the massage rooms, but I fail. We sit in silence while all four of our massage therapists apply powdered Indian sandalwood, one of the most sacred herbs of ayurveda, on our foreheads. This application is used for medicinal and spiritual purposes, which include bringing its recipient closer to the Divine.

"I don't even know what happened in there," Tatiana mumbles, head down, visibly shocked from her massage. I nod in a show of solidarity. From this day on, there is little

Tatiana could ever do wrong. For I will always remember the way she came to be with me here, in India, which goes far beyond the call of sisterly duty. But even beyond that, I will always remember (and she will remind me) how I subjected her to *this*—a spa day where very little spa-ing was had.

Our second chance at another authentic, stress-reducing Indian experience comes a few days later when Dr. Shroff announces she has hired a yoga instructor to teach classes in the physio room.

"Three times a week, Rohit will come to lead yoga. Free to patients and their families. This is for the body *and* the mind!" she shares with excitement one day downstairs. I feel like she is looking straight at me.

Yoga, a gentle practice originating in India, seems so apropos for my healing. I have taken occasional classes at home before, never falling madly in love with it, but perhaps I just haven't found the right class for me. Everyone I know who does yoga, looooves yoga. Yoga is not just an activity, it's a way of life. Based on the people I know, once yoga finds you, you don't just "go" to yoga or "do" yoga. You *become* it. I want this, but my natural personality and patience levels are not well matched to an activity that requires great focus, long periods of time, and resistance to distractions. Still, I am willing to try again in India, convinced it will be more magical here.

Tatiana and I head to our first class, armed with sisterly strength and a huge dose of ambition. Our teacher, Rohit, is instantly easy to read. He's all about the practice and absolutely not about any fun. He is standing in front of class wearing a black shirt, gray sweatpants, and black socks pulled up over them. He looks like he is ready to wade through us, a sea of inexperienced newbies, and transform us into serious yogis.

Rohit begins. He directs us to perform impossible moves as if he's forgotten we are beginners—and disabled. My body rattles while I try to hold it in place, stay focused on my breath, and not fall flat on my face. I can't stop staring at Rohit's socks (*Why are they so high? And why is it more important to me than downward dog?*), but I suspect it's all a game in my brain trying to tease me into useless distraction. I press on and refocus my attention, only to find myself counting sweat drops that fall from my forehead. I am failing all attempts at being disciplined. When I insist to Rohit that I can't bend the way he is directing us—actually, none of us can, which is why we're here—he expects nothing less than for me to at least "try, try!" He waits for me until I attempt the pose, and miserably fail in front of the large mirrored wall. I am panting like a Saint Bernard less than eight minutes in. Tatiana is next to me, doing as he says, face forward, terrified to be caught communicating with the class troublemaker.

"Keep working on your breath. Breeeeaaathe makes miracles," he says repeatedly as he walks past me, eyes fix-ated.

I desperately want to be one of those students who feels transformed on the mat, won't miss a class, and makes my master proud. Instead, I find my mind wandering and my eyes locked on the clock, daydreaming of fleeing the building for shopping at the markets instead. Still, I go to class each day and I *try, try!* as if my life depends on it. I am determined to find the joy everyone else does in this practice. My classmates are reenergized in the halls after our sessions. Even Tatiana seems to have wrangled herself into acceptance of it after a few classes. I want to be in love with yoga. I want to *be* yoga.

Seven days later, after Tatiana has left India, I am back in class, alone in the country and on this mat. That's when I have a very real epiphany. I remember when I was eight years old and my mom made me finish a torturous year of Girl Scouts, even though I hated it, to honor my com-mitment. As I got older, I forced myself to finish reading books I'd started no matter how much I disliked them. And I start to think about how I always force myself to fol-low through when I want to quit, say yes to things when I want to say no, and push myself when I need to rest.

This is what I get clear about: My problem is not and has never been struggling to do the right thing, the good thing, the disciplined thing. My problem has been doing those things whatever the cost to me. I am tired of *try, try!*, of doing things only because they are good for me or because I should, of trying to make things feel *great* when they are not. I have always been so hard on myself—my own harshest critic, rigid judge, and sharpest punisher.

One Wednesday morning, with my last perfect breath of the class, I give myself permission to exit yogaland gracefully. I do it without any of my normal decision-making agony or guilt. Life, like yoga, is all about being okay with exactly where you are. And, as a greeting card from my sister, Lauren, says, it's also about trying not to fart.

Based on those parameters, I decide I have mastered enough of this practice. I pick up my mat and roll it up. I duck out when it's over, proud and calm, but mostly relieved that for the rest of my trip, I can breathe any damn way I want.

I leave the room knowing I will not return. While other patients continue to file into the sweaty yoga sessions, I will practice the act of honoring myself. I do not want to waste another minute obsessing over Rohit's wardrobe choices or studying the tiny scratch on the face of the wall clock. I do not love yoga. I do not want to *be* yoga. I want to bail. For me, learning to say no is what I really need.

I strut out of the building directly into the polluted air of the city. It is particularly quiet in that moment, and I am acutely aware of how untethered Delhi is to any kind of consistency. Just when I think I know what to expect, I see that I don't. This city is not owned or obligated. It is perfectly anarchic. It is a city that helps me say no to my own set of rules and regulations; and encourages me to be whoever I am in each and every moment.

What I need now, and what I want now, is to give myself permission to get off the mat, and take the life that is waiting for me.

8

When You Know, You Know

I am lying facedown in a hunter-green gown on a long, narrow table. Huge round lights that hang from the ceiling are glowing over my body. My arrival at Dr. Shroff's other hospital in Gautam Nagar came after a wild ride through the city and ended in a dusty alleyway blooming with brightly dressed children at play, wandering dogs, and men pushing carts full of papayas. I have been moved to Gautam Nagar because the Green Park hospital doesn't have an operating theater.

A heater is blowing gentle warmth into my face while three medical assistants stand at attention by my side. I am shocked to see that one of them is the handsome, cheerful O.P., who picked us up at the airport almost two months ago. Apparently, he is a jack-of-all-trades. I balance my happiness at seeing him against the sobering fact that my airport greeter is going to help during my surgery. I am relieved to find out that *this* is his real job. Picking up patients from the airport is only something he does in his downtime.

Dr. Ashish enters the room wearing the universal operating room attire: baggy mint-colored scrubs and a surgical mask that covers most of his face. I can see the smiling expression in his eyes. He's completely relaxed as always, but looks even more so since he's not in his usual dress pants and button-up shirt.

It's time for my big moment, my grand finale—The Procedure. The Procedure is a common term around Nutech and refers to the injection of millions of embryonic stem cells directly into the spine.

The hospital is always abuzz with talk about who is getting The Procedure and when. This way of administering stem cells is highly coveted because patients often see dramatic results afterward: a notable boost in strength, moving fingers or toes that didn't move before, and increased stamina. It is mostly used for patients with spinal cord injuries in order to direct the stem cells directly to the area of injury. But once in a while, Dr. Shroff and Dr. Ashish will have another type of patient they think could benefit, and schedule them for one. Today, I am one of those lucky ones!

Even though all of us are so grateful for each and every stem cell we receive, it's hard to avoid being greedy about tomorrow's dose. When it comes to stem cells, there is never too much of a good thing. We discuss treatment schedules, comparing who gets what and when, and are disappointed when we hear that someone else has gotten more than us. We are kids on Halloween night sizing up our sacks of candy. To a stem cell junkie, The Procedure is an overflowing plastic pumpkin bucket full of extra-large chocolate bars.

Dr. Shroff and Dr. Ashish are not sure exactly how much the Procedure will help me, if at all. What they hope it will do is empower my lower body even more before I leave in less than two weeks. But since I'm the first Lyme disease patient they've actually treated, we never really *know* what my reaction to any of the treatment protocols will be. This is something I try not to think of too often.

My pink-and-orange-striped fleece pajama pants are pulled down, midbutt. Dr. Ashish tilts the operating table so my head and upper torso are tipped down toward the floor. The table now feels more like a balance beam than anything else. I double-check with Dr. Ashish that I won't slide forward—and off. "No no!" he says, laughing. I wonder if I'm the only one worried about this. One of the sisters places her hand on my butt to secure me, and I convince myself that, if she had to, she could catch me by one cheek if I should slip.

Dr. Ashish feels intently for the right spot in my spine and injects a local anesthetic at my tailbone. It hurts, but I know it will be over soon. A few minutes go by and the anesthesia sets in. I am remarkably calm, but one clear thought does cross my mind: *Is it okay to let them do this?* I once had a test done at home where fluid was removed from my spine to be analyzed, but maybe I should be more cautious about allowing someone to put something *into* it? In another country? Where we don't know how I'll react?

The thoughts of panic are too late as I start to feel a deep ache and an intense pulling in my lower back. I wince, and Dr. Ashish tells me he is pushing the first syringe full of stem cells into my spine. It's happening! I can't see his hand, but I feel his arm is steady as an iron rod. I breathe deeply, eyes closed, while I try to inhale the new cells into me.

I feel them being infused. A weighted sensation quickly coats my sacrum. If I knew what it was like to have a gorilla sitting on me, I imagine it would feel like this. I wiggle my toes to comfort myself. I know nothing is wrong, but the feeling is so strange that I want to check that everything still works. A lot of my new friends at the hospital are paralyzed, and I think about them now. I came here feeling my legs and I want to leave the same way.

Pressure rises up my spine as the second syringe of

stem cells is slowly injected. I imagine the red line in an old-fashioned thermometer heating up rapidly. But it soon stabilizes and holds still in one place, about halfway up my rib cage. I am giving Dr. Ashish a play-by-play of what I'm feeling as he explains what he's doing.

"Good, good," he keeps repeating. "Verrrrry good."

My right leg and foot start to tingle as the stem cells reach them. "My left leg doesn't feel quite the same as the right one," I report to Dr. Ashish. He slowly tips the table to the left, and almost instantly, that side floods with equal sensations. I imagine my spinal cord now evenly coated with stem cells, thick like molasses. Gauze is placed on the injection area, and it is over.

Within minutes, O.P. helps me roll over onto my back and moves me to a gurney. As we pass through the double doors that lead to the tiny gated elevator, I am totally and completely overwhelmed with emotion—pure contentment. I look up to see a sign that reads LABOR AND DELIVERY and remember how this hospital was originally home to Dr. Shroff's infertility practice. It is the right place for new beginnings.

From my recovery room, I hear kids running and jumping in the school playground next door. The sound of their laughter is louder than the traffic. The purple curtains swing in the light breeze. It is finally warm enough to have the windows open.

Bricks have been placed under the foot of my bed to keep the top half of my body tipped down toward the floor, mimicking the position I was in on the operating table. "We lower your head toward the floor," O.P. explains, "so that gravity will help some of the stem cells to travel toward your brain." *It could use all the help it can get at this point*, I think. O.P.'s final words before he leaves are: "Stay like this for five hours, and then we will slowly lift you."

Within one hour, I have to pee and my appetite is raging.

The TV is small and far away from the bed, so I don't bother asking any of the sisters to turn it on. There are no English channels or Internet at this hospital, not that I'd be in a position to enjoy them anyway.

When Dr. Shroff comes to visit a couple of hours later, I beg her for food. "I will send something," she says. A few minutes later, I am lying flat on my back, but am somehow managing to funnel my favorite spinach chicken and yellow dal into my mouth. I am now not just *eating* Indian food; I am devouring it. This is a contact sport. Sauce drips from the corners of my mouth onto my gown, but I don't ease up.

Five hours go by s-l-o-w-l-y before I am finally allowed to turn on my side for an hour. Once I conquer that with no dizziness, I am allowed to sit up. After I do that successfully, I have completed all phases of The Procedure. The only thing to do next is let it work.

It is after dark when I'm driven back to Green Park, my lower back achy and still bandaged up. No position that I choose feels comfortable, but I try to focus hard on all the potential of my new stem cells. I imagine them as sparks that are igniting throughout my entire body, celebrating my last hurrah of healing here.

I cannot believe that I will be departing Delhi soon. I am the same person who arrived here and yet am so vastly different. The pounds of heaviness have been lifted from my being and bright new light has flooded into me. India has done this for me as I think only India could. Because it is here that I've learned it is possible to be free wherever I am. I am by no means perfect at this, but perfection too is something I am learning to be free from.

I search for some way to express my deepest gratitude to all who helped make this happen. How can I thank my two doctors here in India for this experience? How can I repay this country that shook me to the core but still didn't let me crack? How can I express gratitude to my parents, my family, and my friends who said "you've got this" when I wasn't sure that I did? And finally, what do I say to my own spirit, which helped me survive this when it felt so impossible? The answer comes to me: I can live. I can leave India and I can just live.

Dr. Shroff has suggested I return in six months for a booster treatment of stem cells, and I cling to this. Although I'll be here for only three weeks next time, I find some solace in knowing I'll be back. This is not something I expected I'd feel, especially when I think back to being that girl who refused Indian food, couldn't get through the day without tears, and thought every whiff of smoke in India meant that there was a fire.

I have become attached to this city now—its kind souls, the simplicity of my life here, and the spark of myself that I feel walking through the streets, even in the face of some very harsh realities. I might even go as far as to say I'll miss *everything* here—well, everything except the overzealous honking of endless horns.

The truth is, I am also afraid to go home. I am afraid because going home means having to embrace the complexities of life once again. Here, my home is my tiny hospital room, my food is already chosen, my friends are built-in, and my life is self-contained in this neighborhood. There are no big questions about life to answer, no grand plans to be made, and no expectations to rise to.

I am also worried about being without these daily injections of stem cells. I have spent years challenging a disease that, despite some triumphs, has left me always wondering what will be. It's ironic that no matter what is going on, whether good or bad, I always feel I'm a stranger to my future.

In spite of missing India and wondering what will follow my departure, I am also grateful to be near the end of my stay. I want to brush my teeth with tap water, know my clothes will come out perfectly clean after being washed, and see the faces of those at home I love so much. There is nothing I want more than to kiss Zach's plump little cheeks until he screams.

The last weeks here in Delhi become like the last week of the school year—when you can't focus on work, because the fun things are constantly calling your attention away. I spend every minute I can out at the lively markets, strolling through the broken-up paths of Hauz Khas, and gathering my last moments in the city's playground.

The *feeling* of health is still with me the week before my departure. It is still with me, because now, it *is* me.

Two days before my flight home I begin to pack, but it is the kind of packing where you just shift things around so it feels like you are doing something, even though nothing is happening. It doesn't matter to whom or what I have had to say good-bye; I am not good at it. I think maybe ever since Poppy died, I've been allergic to good-byes.

The hardest good-bye I ever said was the day in 2007, only one year earlier, when I said it to Jay. It was one of the biggest, scariest, leaping decisions of my life.

Despite my reluctance, Jay and I had recently bought a house with the generous help of my parents, and, to go with that new house, had adopted an adorable but wildly untrained four-month-old Rottweiler puppy. Because when things are already hard, I like to complicate them even further. Every day of that first summer in our new home, we lounged by the pool and sipped beer on the patio, watching the pink sunsets over the mountains behind our house. We painted the grand wall in the living room pinot noir red and hung a giant flat-screen on the wall. If you were looking in from the outside, it would look like everything was *great*. But the biggest lie that we tell ourselves is that everything is *great*. *It's great! Really, I'm great! Life is great! Our relationship is great!* We can lie to other people for a long, long time, but the clock on lying to ourselves runs out a whole lot faster.

The real story was this.

It had taken a long few months after the infamous "you're fine now" Mayo Clinic trip to realize that no amount of physical therapy was going to cure me, no matter how intent I was on making it so. I was still sick. The pain and weakness was a slightly lesser version of before, but only thanks to a new medication. I could drive myself. I was gardening when I could. And I was living some kind of life, even though what I had been through, and was still going through, made my entire world feel like I was trudging through thick mud.

It was not only breaking Jay and me individually, but our relationship too. What had started as warning signals that we weren't going to last had now become giant flashing neon signs. It was officially clear that the couple built on fun was not made for the life we had. He was telling me less and less about his life, and shutting me out more. I was doing the same. Sometimes we'd sit and watch TV and I could feel his resentment just billowing toward me. He made little comments and digs, and it was obvious that he wasn't happy. Sometimes it was more pronounced when he drank, but it was always there. One night while Jay and I were walking home from our neighborhood bar, he deliberately and forcefully shoved his shoulder into mine. It wasn't an accident and he didn't offer an apology. As I stumbled and then recovered, he just kept walking. When I asked him why he did that, he begrudgingly said that I was in the way.

Maybe his angst toward me had been there from the start, covered up most of the time with the fun we used to have; and maybe it had only grown with all we had been through, a life that he never signed up for. We tried to hit reset all the time, with date nights and promises of better communication; but our attempts almost always ended up in fights and more misery no matter what we did. The more we seemed to fall apart, the harder I pushed myself to be more perfect—I made sophisticated meals, tried to be more fun and spontaneous, and acted unbothered by the upsetting things he did or said. Maybe I did this in order to fix us or maybe it was to ensure that whatever happened to us wouldn't be my fault.

What I eventually discovered is that there are two ways that human beings move on from things that our souls know we need to be finished with. Either, a) we go of our own accord, making decisions that rise from deeply centered conviction and confidence; or, b) we go kicking and screaming, because despite all signs that point us to the viable option of going gracefully, we can only go when we *have* to go.

But I had mostly only known one way my whole life, and this time was no exception. If I had acted on any of my gut feelings about leaving Jay before then, it would have been some version of going gracefully. But I did not act on them, because at that point, I was convinced that I didn't know what to do.

"If you don't know, *you know*. Just trust your gut. It's that simple," my always sensible brother once told me when I begged him for relationship advice. But for me, it wasn't simple. "I don't know" had become a very good cop-out in my life, and an escape from many things: making hard decisions, hurting people's feelings, and having to figure out what was way down inside. *Ignore and it does not exist. Everything is great.*

I have always loved the idea of *trust your gut* and *you already know*. But what do you do when your gut is so damn good at hiding everything from you? I realize now that I probably always did have the answers. I was just not yet ready to tell myself the truth. Because telling yourself the truth is hard, but acting on your truth is even harder.

Jay and I had each been to therapists in the past, but we'd never gone together. So when Jay suggested we go to couples therapy, I agreed, even though I think a part of me recognized that it would only prolong what was already on the horizon.

Diane, our middle-aged and cheery therapist, spent the first five minutes of each session telling us about the joys of new motherhood with her adopted baby boy. In our sessions, I'd complain about Jay, he'd complain about me, and Diane would help us complain in a productive way. Using a ball of yarn, she would make circles around each of us, marking visual spaces in which we could safely express ourselves. I held back tears and struggled to speak my mind, sometimes waiting all week to say things I could only do with the safety of Diane and my circle of yarn. "Nothing I do ever seems good enough for him. . . . I'm just not the person he wants me to be. . . . It feels like he gets mad at me for everything, and is resentful toward me for being sick."

Jay, when prompted by Diane to respond, would always be loving, understanding, and sexily self-aware. Nothing pairs with a bad boy better than emotional intelligence.

Listening to him talk about us always made me doubt my own feelings. "But remember how much fun we had at the zoo last weekend?" he'd ask me, the question tinted with amnesia. And "Things really aren't *that* bad. There are still many more good times than bad," he'd assure Diane. If our relationship were a trip to the county fair and each of us were asked to recount our experience of it, I'd remember the whole picture, including the exorbitant cost and long, arduous lines. Jay would remember only the thrill of the rides.

About two months into our adventures in couples therapy, Jay got stuck at work and couldn't make it to our session. I decided to go anyway. I heard about the new words Diane's baby boy had mumbled that week ("Mama! Ba ba! No!"). When she asked me how things were going, I told her the more transparent version of what I said every week in front of Jay. "I'm not happy. . . . I can't be myself with him. . . . I love him and am so thankful for all he's done, but this just doesn't fit."

"I have to tell you . . . you are playing the victim," Diane said matter-of-factly as I sat alone on her couch made for two. "You know, you don't have to stay," she went on. "Every week you're upset by the same types of things, and rightfully so. But this is who Jay is, and if things aren't changing, you don't have to stay. You get to *go*."

I was stunned into silence and a little bit angry. *This*

isn't my fault! I'm the sick one, the hurt one, I thought. *It's not that easy to go!*

Playing the victim. Diane's comment sank into me over the next few days. I didn't know exactly what it meant, but I somehow felt her words as a secret truth of mine. I knew in my heart that we really didn't fit, and I really did want to go. But a voice was screaming *Not now!* in my head.

He's been so supportive. *Not now.*

He's my best friend. *Not now.*

It's not his fault. *Not now.*

He can't help who he is. *Not now.*

You are sick. *Not now.*

He loves your family. *Not now.*

Maybe things really aren't *that* bad. *Not now.*

A week after my solo appointment with Diane, the tension in our house was combustible. The things that were already bad got worse. The pressure I felt to get better, to save our relationship, to be the person Jay wanted me to be, was breaking me. Then one day a series of events unfolded in such a perfectly disastrous way that all my wavering disappeared.

Based on some hunches and other terrible feelings that drove me to become that crazy person I never wanted to be, I became heroically stronger than Jay's password-setting skills and broke into his e-mail account while he was at work. Not my finest hour, I know. I looked through this window into his life with a sinking stomach. What I saw was not the loyal Jay I knew.

And for the first time ever, something inside of me whispered, *Now, now.*

I called only three people when I decided to leave. These are the people you call when you sound the alarm for your own life—these are your "fire people."

"Daddy, I have to go. What should I do?"

"Call Jay at work and tell him," he said. And then, "Come and stay with us, baby." I heard my mom next to him, trying to figure out what was going on. It felt like my parents, who now lived nine hours away, were on the other side of the world.

"Melissa, please come help me pack."

Melissa and I have been friends since we were twelve years old. She makes the best funny faces, but appears in two seconds with all seriousness if you ever need her in a crisis. About a year before this, Melissa had called me to help her with some rescue kittens she took in. "I know this is gross," she said when I arrived, holding up cotton balls in one hand and a kitten in the other, "but we have to stimulate their anal glands." Even though we laughed through it, I promised I'd get her back one day. So when I called her, I think she was comforted to find out it was only to pack.

"Jay, I have to go."

This was the hardest call, because he was still one of my fire people and also my best friend. All he said was "Okay, Ames" in a quiet monotone voice. I thought I heard relief, but I didn't question it.

There were things I always knew about our relationship and things I never knew. I always knew that Jay had the most tender, loving, sensitive heart. I always knew how I deeply loved him. I also knew, although it took me a long time to realize, that the hurtful things Jay said and did were not my fault. Like me, he had his own cracks.

What I never knew was that none of that mattered.

I never knew that there was only one thing to know, which was that I couldn't be *me* around *him*. It didn't matter why that was true; just that it was. And I never knew that while someone might be your very best friend, the person you love, and the person that you really really *really* wish fit, you might still have to go.

Melissa and I packed only what could fit in my supercool vanilla Dodge Magnum, which Jay had helped me trade for my not-so-cool green Ford Explorer. Then I explained to the dog why I couldn't stay. Bob, with his sad Rottweiler eyes and his stout stature, stood there, ears back, whining as I closed the door behind myself. Making the decision to go is hard, calling your fire people is big, but the moment of truth actually comes when you tell the dog.

I made it only two hours north in my overpacked car before I realized the hugeness of my decision and couldn't drive anymore. I stopped at a hotel, checked into a cozy fireplace room, and climbed into bed with my shattered heart. It was 6 p.m.

I cried until my eyes ran dry. I called my parents. I tried to avoid texting Jay, which I was not so great at, so I locked my phone in the glove compartment of my car. I took a bath, wishing for it to wash away my old life.

The next morning I continued on to Mendocino, another six hours up the California coast. I can't tell you how I got there, though, because it seemed like the car just drove itself. Surely I helped, but I don't recall any actual details of the road or other cars. I think I was still wearing my pajamas. I pulled the car over every so often to get out, perch myself on the edge of the forest that met the road, and dispel my anxiety through my tears. The dampness in the air matched the density of grief in my lungs.

Even though parts of me ached more deeply than ever before, I could feel that part of my healing was in the leaving.

I have that same feeling now, crouched on the dirty floor of my hospital room, cramming my belongings into three dusty suitcases. India has become an unexpected safe haven that now feels like home. But if I want to grow into a new life, I cannot stay suspended in this temporary one.

The zipper on my largest case is busting open, even as I try to sit on top to contain it. It quickly becomes clear that there is not enough room inside for all the belongings from my new life.

What I have collected includes: enough Ganesha and elephant figurines to open my own shop, several packets of Indian spices, a plethora of bangles I was told (after my proud purchase) certainly contain toxic lead, and a few dresses that I couldn't say no to.

I also have drugs. Lots of drugs.

Over the years, I've gotten accustomed to needles, nasty-tasting pills, and messy powdered concoctions. But what I've never quite gotten accustomed to is the *MUST PAY CASH* notes when I pick up my prescriptions at the pharmacy. More often than not, my insurance doesn't think I need these medications, even though my doctors do.

In India, these same prescriptions cost about a third of what I pay in the US. And the pharmacy delivers to my room for free. I have taken several different antibiotics here while we try to figure out what's best for my body and the stem cells. This is likely to continue for some time at home, so I'm leaving with everything I might need . . . and I'm taking it for a bargain.

At home, I fork over $500 each month for a common antibiotic called Zithromax. Here, the exact same brand and dosage comes in just shy of $14. The IV antibiotic I've been receiving in India costs more than $70 a day at home. Here, it costs $5.

I feel a driving urge to take requests from Lyme-disease-sabotaged friends back home and even new friends following my blog. I want to bring candy-colored pills and liquids to all in need. If US Customs would let me, I could be the Santa of sick people, bearing a tiny reprieve from one of the challenges of managing uncontrollable, chronic disease. In this cost-effective country, I am so overjoyed at my "found" money, I almost lose sight of the unfairness of having to take home all this medicine in the first place.

I decide the only way to deal with this packing crisis is to ditch one of my medium-size suitcases and get a brand-new, larger one to take home.

I hit the streets, which are, as always, bubbling with action. Delhi's winter has finally passed, and even though it's not officially summer yet, it's hot enough to make me sweat. The sisters have put away the blankets in their nursing stations and are now using hand fans to stay cool.

I make my way down the road, past a man selling coconut water, around a corner where a woman begs for rupees, down another street full of children playing cricket, over a center divider where a giant black cow is lounging, through a pungent food market, and finally over two more lanes of insane traffic.

That's when I see a luggage shop with every size and

type I could ever need: rolling suitcases, duffel bags, and backpacks galore. They are spilling out onto the broken dirt paths that barely resemble sidewalks, and passersby are kicking dust on them.

Examining my choices, I find one with a sticker made from masking tape. This is *my* bag—a new container for my new life. It reads: 2XL.

I name it Big Blue 2XL and buy it for a bargain.

Heading back to the hospital, I decide to take a new route, even though I'm not totally sure it's even really a route back at all. Instead of sidewalks, huge ditches run along the storefronts, allowing only an extremely narrow path beyond to walk on. And I now have an enormous suitcase to balance. It must be lunch hour because it seems everyone in the city is on this street with me. There is no room to carry my new purchase by my side. It is now clear why Indians carry things on their heads: bowls, food, bundles of sticks, you name it. If you don't, you risk getting knocked down, tipped over, and pushed against a car.

When in Rome . . . I flip the suitcase up onto my head, one arm strapped around each side, and begin to make my way back to the hospital. I revel at my awesome balance, my confidence in navigating the streets, and my ability to perform both these tricky tasks with ease. I hear deep belly laughs from some of the locals as I walk through the streets. Turning, I see I am actually faring almost as well as the lady next to me, who is carrying a huge pile of produce on her head. I can only imagine what I look like: white skin, long blond curly hair, pink lip gloss, oversize sunglasses, and a gigantic suitcase on my head.

When I get closer to the hospital, I cut through the back alley. A dog in a sweater sleeps at the entrance of a hidden Hindu temple, children throw peanuts at each other, and a monkey skips through the crowds. That is when I hear *the voice*. It's *him*. His prayers are echoing through the air clearer than I've ever heard them before. It is only one more minute before I see my guru with the megaphone. He is younger than I imagined, clean-shaven with slicked-back hair, and is gliding on a black bicycle with crooked handlebars.

I can finally understand some of his words. I keep reciting the first part over and over so I don't forget it—*"Aum shreem hreem kleem klowm gum . . ."*—but the rest dissipates into the chaos around me. He turns my way with his dark chestnut eyes and offers the start of a smile, as if he knows me in the same way that I know him. It's the last time I will ever hear his voice.

I will later learn that these words I have come to love are from the Maha Ganapati Mool chant. This chant is used to invoke Lord Ganesha, the elephant-headed god, the remover of obstacles. It is chanted before beginning new projects as a way to remove obstacles and aid in the success of one's efforts.

Out alone in dusty Delhi, I feel fear and freedom simultaneously. This mystical land has pushed me to the brink of insanity, but has also carried me into the depths of a love I've never known. It has been both everything I despise and exactly what I have needed. Without India's insistence that I survive it, I am stagnant, safe, like a boat hugging the shore and wasting my sails.

The obstacles of this life are plentiful, but so too are the opportunities to find peace. I feel this out in the city, but even more so in the wild uncertainty of my own unsteady heart.

With the suitcase on my head and this new life before me, I ask myself, *How does it feel to be on my own?*

The answer that comes surprises me.

It feels *necessary*.

9

Yes

My return home from India in February 2008 will be one of both rapturous joy and absolute uncertainty. Lauren has offered something that only the most generous of sisters would: for me to move in with her, Craig, and Zach in Monterey Bay, California, a city by the sea. I accept gladly. Zach is now a full-fledged toddler, and he and I make up for lost time by doing everything together. We visit playground after playground and have deep conversations over sushi about why restaurants make their tablecloths white. I can run multiple errands at once without getting fatigued. I don't trip when walking on uneven terrain. I don't trip at all. I take only a few medications. I feel free as a bird.

I will also survive a handful of lows—medical tests that shake my confidence, reminding me I'm not invincible; coming face-to-face with fears about my life and my future; and continuing to struggle with being patient and kind to myself, which still doesn't come so easily. The doctors think that I'm likely over Lyme, but still consider me an experiment. No one knows what to do with me or how to ensure I'll retain all the improvements I've gained.

In July, almost six months after I left, I return to India—my beloved nemesis and best teacher. Both the hospital and I look different. The lobby has gotten a serious face-lift—modern black faux-leather chairs have replaced the old wooden furniture, and the rickety reception desk has been upgraded to a sleek modern one that is double the size. As for me, my hair is a new and darker shade of blond and I am now comfortable wearing only minimal makeup. I have also gained twenty healthy pounds since my first trip here, which does not go unnoticed. "I like this. I reaaaally like this!" O.P. keeps repeating through his sparkly teeth. The sisters run toward me, spin me around like a doll, and puff out their little cheeks. "You look fattened!" Sahana shrieks, then quickly follows with, "This sooooo niiiiice!"

In many ways, this trip echoes the first. I take more antibiotics to protect my cells, my emotional and physical stability is sometimes questionable, and India continues to teach me my greatest lesson—that every day is a swinging pendulum between saving your life and enjoying it. It also delivers added improvements: clearer cognitive abilities (I finally have the concentration to read an entire book!), less light and sound sensitivity, more strength, and increased endurance.

When I bid my last farewell three weeks later at Indira Gandhi International Airport, I intend to let my ten-year visa lapse and never choke on the city's pollution again. It is a chapter closed. But the assumption that I have kissed India good-bye for a final time only proves my stupidity. If there is anything India has shown me, it is that it will do with me what it pleases.

The remainder of the year is a heady mix of emotions and adjustments. I have no real place in the world. Everything needs to be re-created. I can see so far ahead, and yet not anything at all. Sometimes I revel in the freedom of being able to float without direction . . . there is nothing to do or be right now. But then the vast emptiness of it becomes luminous and scares me.

Instead of allowing this emptiness to intimidate me, I decide to say yes to filling the space of it. I think that's how rebuilding is done. So it's exactly what I do: I start saying yes.

My first *yes* comes during my birthday month of September when I drive back toward the life I ran away from and ask Jay to join me in attempting some version of closure. It doesn't feel right to close this chapter on illness without letting him close it too. We head back to my favorite town of Ojai, with its abundant trees and rose-colored sunsets; and the place where I believe I was bitten by that tiny tick. Since our breakup, the strain and sorrows between us have been heavy; so much so that we hardly spoke while dividing up our belongings and differences. But on this day, as we stare at the deep, sprawling crevices of a strong and sturdy symbolic oak tree, it is all unity. Jay photographs the moment and cheers while I sprint around it, as many times as I can, leaping over bushes with an energy all its own. Bob bounces behind me the way dogs do, unsure of what he's celebrating but joining in for the pure love of it. I see Jay wipe his eyes behind the camera as I stomp all of those unpleasant memories back into the earth, as hard as I can, and put them to rest.

My next *yes* comes in December 2008, a year after my first trip to India, when Dr. Harr asks if he can test me again to see if I am now Lyme disease–free. "Yes!" I say. The test comes back after two long weeks of waiting, and when it does, it replies, "No." *No, you are not clear. No, you are not perfect.* The test is positive for Lyme disease. And even though all the doctors tell me not to panic, I do. They explain to me that sometimes this happens when your body finally recognizes a disease and is fighting it. This could even be a good thing, they reassure me. But the panic isn't because I may not be free of Lyme disease. The panic is because I have to *tell this* to a lot of people—all the people in my life and all the people following my story and my blog. I want to hide this new information, let nobody see me naked in this way, and bury the test results very far down somewhere deep in the ground. But instead, I do the opposite. I tell people. I write it on my blog. I bare my soul. I say yes to *being human*, and doing it publicly. It's the hardest thing I've ever done in my whole life and will take much practice for me to become comfortable with it. But what I realize at this point is that maybe I'm not destined to be a Lyme disease superhero or a stem cell poster child or any kind of inspirational figure at all. Maybe I'm here for what we're all here for: to show each other that it's okay to be human.

Next it is time to say yes to the fact that adjusting to being healthy is harder than I thought it would be. This is all I've wanted, yet the feat of rejoining a world that I've missed out on for so many years is overwhelming. *How can I catch up now? What's next? How will I get a job again with such a huge gap in my work history? Where will I live when I move out of my sister's guest room? How will I ever afford it? Can I find a partner who will accept all of me?* I want to stretch out completely into the world, yet I am still tied to a brain that's acclimated only to a life of illness. The doctors' voices are in my head, telling me not to get stressed or catch a cold or the flu, because it could cause me to relapse—a common occurrence with Lyme patients. *Am I safe? Can I enjoy this luxury and freedom of my improved health? Will it all slip away when I'm off having fun and not looking? What if it happens again? What if it is already happening again and I just don't know it yet?* I am always either afraid of life with illness, or afraid of life without it.

But I think it's important to look at every stretch of time in our lives as a whole, and to identify how we feel *most* about it, *most* of the time. When I add up everything that happens during this stretch of time after India, including when things aren't total perfection, I can still identify my primary feeling about it: thankful.

My final *yes* for 2008 comes when I am asked to speak about my stem cell experience to a roomful of resident doctors at Stanford University. All eyes are on me in my high heels (yeehaw . . . heels without tripping!), tight jeans, and silk button-up top. With the lights above me humming, my nerves take over and I forget the opening line of my speech. What comes out of my mouth instead is this: "I wish you could have seen me one year ago today." It is this moment that will kick off a grant project, created to study the benefits of stem cell treatment in Lyme disease patients. While the grant will never end up being funded and approved, the invitation to work on the project will take me back to India the following year for one final *yes*.

It is during my third trip to India in March 2009, full of street smarts and feeling like a native, that I convince myself it's perfectly fine to eat a succulent tandoori shrimp lunch from a food cart. It turns out I do not have the stomach of a native. When I am predictably struck down with Delhi belly, I am forced to extend my trip for another five days, staying at Nutech Mediworld at the insistence of Dr. Shroff. This city was not done with me yet.

A few days later, down in the physio room, I am finally just a visitor and no longer a patient. It's there, amid the loud Hindi music that is beating through my entire body, that I see Charlotte for the first time. Her brown curly locks are peeking out from under a Kelly green baseball cap. She is visiting her mother, Janet, a sweet British woman I had met while recouping at the hospital. Janet is around fifty years old, and almost doll-like, with fair skin, pink cheeks, and lilac-painted fingernails. She has ALS (Lou Gehrig's disease) and is here hoping these stem cells are the miracle she needs. For the past few mornings, I have been visiting with her as she excitedly counts down to Charlotte's arrival. Janet adores Charlotte and has promised me that I too will fall in love with her. She paints a dreamy picture of us jaunting through the city together, lunching, and forming a fabulous friendship.

Charlotte is magnetic, quirky, and energetic, a film trailer editor from London with the most brilliant British accent. Whatever she says automatically sounds a hundred times more special because of the way she says it. And just as Janet predicted, I actually *do* want to lunch with her.

She is the wittiest person I've ever met. She is so funny that when she makes me laugh, I involuntarily throw my head back. We go on adventures each day together, for three days in a row. Sometimes it's just for tea. Sometimes it's to wander the streets, where we see random peacocks or cows, and discuss the hopes and horrors of India. When she comes back to my hospital room to hang out, I ask her to take her shoes off. I want her to stay awhile. Charlotte is not just a new person to me, but a whole new *kind* of person to me. As I learn more about her, I only become more enthralled. Her latest work project is *Mamma Mia*, she lives in an old match factory in east London, she's gay, *The Sound of Music* is pretty much her favorite thing ever, and she loves the smell of fresh cut grass. I have never even noticed the smell of fresh cut grass. I find out that she already knows about me, because she has been following my blog. Which means she already knows I'm *human*. I can't decide how I feel about this, but it's too late anyway.

On our last evening together before I go home, Charlotte and I sit on the steps of the hospital, deep in conversation. I am not sure how I will live without our daily walks and shenanigans. I am also not sure how I have become this intrigued by someone in such a short period of time. I want to never stop seeing her. I want to melt into her.

I am in love with Charlotte.

I sit with this for a moment, but I don't let myself panic.

I tell myself I am probably wrong, even though I know I'm not wrong at all. And then I think, *No, no, I am not wrong. I am in love with Charlotte.* This is perhaps my biggest *yes*, because even though I don't yet tell her what I'm feeling, I say yes to telling myself the truth right when I know it. It is about time.

Charlotte is my *coming home.* It is not because she provides for me what I need in order to be happy or what I cannot provide for myself. It's because she says in every single way, *I accept you.* And this helps me continue to say it to myself. There are no parameters or consequences. We are equals. That is the story that Charlotte tells me about myself. With Charlotte, I want to love with my emotions wide open, even though it is terrifying.

Some of my family and friends are in shock, asking me, "How does it feel to be with a woman?" and sometimes, "Are you totally positive this is what you want?" But the thing is that this feels like nothing out of the ordinary. It is easy and right. Sometimes these questions make me think that I should be concerned and maybe even go to therapy to figure out what this really means about my past relationships and myself. But thankfully, by some miracle, and in a complete deviation from my usual MO, I end up not making this into something it isn't. I don't psychoanalyze the situation. I dig deep for the real feeling inside of me, which is this: It is love. The end. No more discussion. I am not worried, confused, or inquisitive about my sexuality or what this means in the scheme of my entire life or past. Because this is only love. And love, on its own, before we start to pick it apart, is really quite straightforward.

I am visiting Charlotte in London's bitter cold December when the already dark winter dims the lights on us. Janet is home from India and getting weaker despite two trips for stem cells. I visit her during the day while Charlotte is at work, showing her pictures and videos of Zach, who is three, and growing like a weed. Janet can't speak at all now, as the disease has progressed to its final stages. I fill the air with long, drawn-out descriptions of what I plan to make for dinner and stories from back home, trying to distract her from what we all know is coming. The last day of Janet's life feels like when someone is trying to leave a house party, but people keep pulling them back and stalling their departure. She is, unfortunately, not the recipient of the stem cell miracle she had hoped for. No one is ready for her to go, except for her.

It is Christmas Eve and there is snow on the ground when I call my dad from the hospital. Despite his own issues, he is always the person everyone runs to first in any kind of crisis. I think about some of the late nights when I'd called him before: from a road trip I took in high school where I accidentally drove three hours in the wrong direction, from the community college where I took my first night class and couldn't find the classroom, and from my couch when he didn't show up for our weekly date night to watch *ER* (don't worry, he had just fallen fast asleep in the bookstore). I hear his voice and am instantly relieved. Partly because I need my daddy now, and partly because lately he's been struggling more than ever. *I don't know how much longer he can take this*, my mom has messaged me a few times recently. *I feel like he is serious about dying.* And by dying, she means taking his own life, because after decades of dealing with this, taking his own life is what he talks about when he's having a very hard time. *This will pass as it always does*, I have been telling myself while I'm thousands of miles away. But there is always that one thought: *What if it doesn't?*

"I think Janet's gonna die soon, Daddy," I sniffle into the phone, trying to shelter my whimpers from the nurses' station beside me.

"Do you know what it's like when someone dies?" he asks. "I can tell you if you want so you'll be ready." I shake my head no because I can't speak through the knot in my throat, but he feels my answer.

"Death is not bad, baby," he says. "It's usually slow, less dramatic than you'd imagine, and it's one of the coolest things to ever witness—to watch a human being's suffering become peace." These things he tells me are all I need. I am ready. *Death is not bad, baby.*

Shortly after, Janet lets go. That's when I realize that, for maybe the first time ever, I did not do what I have always done: fight against the current of what is, or search around for one more eleventh-hour cure. Instead, I trusted that *death is not bad, baby,* and when she let go, I let go with her.

We bury Janet just days later under sheets of pounding rain and black umbrellas. It feels like the darkest day of winter because she is gone, but also like the verge of summer, because she is free.

I am still in London in the new year of 2010, when I feel the rumbling of an internal earthquake. I begin to have pain and tingling in my feet and waves of fatigue; my heart races, the deep and constant whole-body aches of my past return, and I'm nauseated no matter what I eat. These are the same symptoms that appeared in 2005, at the beginning of my career as a full-time sick person. I'm also having a flare-up of endometriosis, a diagnosis that came long before Lyme. I've already undergone five surgeries for endometriosis, and still survive my menstrual cycles only with narcotic pain medication and trips to the ER.

At first, I try ignoring these signs of my world shaking. *Ignore and it does not exist.* But the earthquake persists. And a few weeks later, because I am finally learning that ignoring things just never works, I go to the doctor. He admits me to the hospital, and after two days of tests releases me with those infamous words: "We don't know how to fix you." After that, I find out that I have an unrelenting case of Epstein-Barr virus, my food allergies have returned, and the complex coinfections that often accompany Lyme disease are back. The Lyme itself is absent—for now—and I am nowhere close to where I once was, but I'm definitely headed in the wrong direction.

This is the elusive relapse I've been running from, even though I refuse to call it that. Because no Lyme was detected, I've convinced myself that it is not a relapse at all. But alas, something has finally caught up to me. My heart falls into my stomach. I am flooded with fear, consumed by overwhelm, and mad as hell. The doctors are worried about what to do for my menstrual cycles that are causing more pain and fatigue with each month, my immune system that is depleted and dysfunctional, and my body as a whole, which is on a rickety trajectory. But there is only one question that I am concerned with right now: *How in the world did I end up back here again?*

•   •   •

Dear Daddy,

It seems silly to write in your obituary guestbook, as if you are reading it. But I can hear you saying, "How the fuck do you know I'm not?" so I'm gonna roll with it. Being without you has been, in some ways, the hardest time of my life. Every time I want advice, I almost pick up the phone to call you. Every time I learn something new, I reach again. Every time I just miss you, I have to figure out another way to make you hear me. Oh, this is going to take a lot of practice. . . .

There were so many things that made you one of the most incredibly special people in the Universe. When you asked someone a question, even just a "How are you?" you asked it with true curiosity. When you did something, you did it well no matter how many hours or repeats it took to get it just right. After you learned something interesting, you couldn't wait to share it. You tinkered with little things none of us would bother with. You reached out to strangers without hesitation. When something was funny, you told the story over and over, laughing with your big belly laugh as if you were experiencing it for the first time. When you loved someone, you told them.

Although I have struggled immensely with hating that you had to suffer so much in your life, tonight I finally came to something that brings me complete peace. Because of, and in between, your times of suffering, you experienced a level of joy that most never even touch. The good days were better than life. When you smiled, it illuminated the entire space around you. And when you loved, you made people feel it better than anyone else I know.

There is no doubt I will continue to miss you every single day, but what you have left me with says more about you than perhaps anything else. I have the most incredibly strong, fun, and loving mother in the world, an example of marriage and love that has made me settle for nothing less, and siblings I could not imagine being without. Life will be different without you in it. But it does not have to be all about what we lost when you left. What I have gained from being your daughter are genuinely the most beautiful gifts of yourself.

And for the times I need a little more of you in my life, I have your beautiful treasured camera, which I will constantly pull out, taking more pictures than any one human might need of a single thing, just to get the right shot.

> *Love,*
> *Your Favorite*

• • •

CHARLOTTE AND I are living together in our waterside apartment in Los Angeles when I write these last words to my dad. It is early 2011, a few days after his death and one week before my mom's sixty-fourth birthday. We decide not to cancel the dinner party we'd planned at her favorite Indian restaurant, because life is still going on and we have to remind each other that we need to go on too.

The day of the birthday dinner, I make a quick run to Hallmark to find the most special birthday card out there—the one that attempts to make up for your husband dying and your kids possibly bawling through your party. When I leave the house and the safety of our family vigil, I feel raw to the real world. The grief of losing a parent feels like far too much to be contained in any human's body. The sadness is coming in currents that pull me under, even though when I sit and do what I always do—identify my primary feeling for every stretch of time—it is still *relieved*. Dad is no longer suffering.

When we head out to the party that evening, on the way to the car I see blackbirds circling high in the sky. I watch them just as they did when they stopped us in our tracks at the Taj Mahal, and again, more recently, when the coroner came to take Dad while the rest of us huddled in the backyard to shield ourselves from the sight. He is gone, but I can feel now that he is also here for it all. Mom stretches her arms out to the sides, as if walking on an invisible balance beam, unconsciously spreading her wings. It feels like the most vibrant pieces of her that went missing when Dad got sick have already begun to return. She is already *going on*.

As for me, I'm still in limbo.

The episode with my health in London has turned out to be a shadow of what used to be, showing up once again. So I am doing more of what I've done before—taking tinctures and supplements—even though it's clear by now that it isn't a very effective long-term solution.

At the same time, my periods are continuing to get worse. Each month brings days so painful that I'm doubled over and can't function. The fatigue is all-consuming and lasting more of each month. My doctors not only worry that this is causing stress *on* my immune system, but they tell me it's a deeper message *from* my immune system. Something is not right. Because the impact of my periods is posing such a risk to my body as a whole, I have decided on something drastic: a procedure called endometrial ablation, which will destroy the lining of my uterus and cure this disease so I never have to face it again.

But there is still the rest of my body to deal with.

While I am not as sick as I once was, I see at this time that I am not healed either. And what I really want, no, *demand*, is to be done with illness and go on with life.

I have trekked halfway around the world, gone to the best experts, drunk every concoction known to man, allowed healers and specialists to place their miraculous hands upon me, and spent hundreds of thousands of dollars that my family so lovingly scraped together for me. I eat organic foods, protect myself from toxins, and am hyperaware of everything and anything that could impact my health. But this has simply not been enough for complete and permanent healing.

This harsh realization leads me to an epiphany so grand that it almost blows my head off: *If treating the body doesn't resolve the problem, then maybe the body alone isn't causing it.* Which means maybe, just maybe, the problem isn't my body . . . it's me?

That's when, from somewhere in my brain, stored in a folder labeled *Come Back to One Day*, those once-resisted words of Dr. Shroff's show themselves to me. The words are lit up. They are on-screen. They are in all caps. They are: *YOU CAN HEAL YOURSELF.* This is no longer just advice from a doctor. These words are truth.

And just like that, I decide I will *try, try!* as Rohit always encouraged me to do. It is time. I put the tinctures, supplements, and medications away. I cancel my planned endometrial surgery. All the treatments have only bought me time. I have to save my own life.

This idea terrifies me—but instead of ignoring it, instead of running away, I *listen.* Because running away—from my feelings and often away from the truth of my life—has to come to an end. It has to come to an end because I finally understand that this is what's been making me sick.

I start with just that, even though it is only the tip of an iceberg that I can't sense the size of. It is enough for the moment. The many things I discover next won't come to me all at once, in a tidy package delivered by the Universe the way I want them. They will come slowly, intermittently, like stops on a train where miles and bends have to be conquered first.

I begin by reading, researching, and soul-searching. The pain of missing my dad is often overwhelming, distracting, deep, and inconsolable. I want him here so badly now, to have conversations about what I'm learning, to ask him what he thinks; but mostly, I want to know if any of what I need to know now is the same thing he was always missing.

What I discover is this: Our physical bodies are the sum of our lives. Our lives are the sum of our thoughts, beliefs, and emotions. When we suppress our emotions, it can create stress on the physical body, causing emotions to show up as physical symptoms. This is how our body communicates with us, by using its very own language.

I also learn that when we change things that aren't working on the inside, the outside will change too. *Yes,* I am thinking. *Yes.* There is no mind, body, and spirit as separate entities. We are all mind-body-and-spirit. I have

mostly come to this conclusion not by some vast willing-
ness to subscribe to it, but by a basic process of elimination.
It's the only truth left.

This is when I begin to see my body as more than the
rebellious, resistant deterrent to my hopes and dreams
that I took it for. My body is the ultimate secret-keeper of
what's going on inside of me. In fact, my body is perhaps
the only bold-faced, consistent truth teller in my life. And
the truth my body has been speaking through all of its
symptoms is this:

*You are not being you, therefore this home is not for you.
Get out. Please leave. You are Goldilocks trying to live a bear's
life. Nothing fits and nothing is working because you are not
a bear. Find the real person who lives here in this body, this
home, and bring her back. Then I will be happy and so will
you. Goldilocks could not live happily ever after until she
found her own place in the world. And neither can you. Find
the real person who lives here in this body, this home, and
bring her back.*

As if someone is slowly unblindfolding me, I begin to
understand *why* I have not been the real me.

I have been afraid of so many things. I'm afraid I'll
never really be well (and that it's not up to me anyway). I
am afraid that I will be totally well (that it's *all* up to me).
I am afraid of trusting myself. I am afraid of making mis-
takes. I'm afraid of people being upset with me. I am afraid

to relax. I'm afraid of my own truth. I am afraid of living in a world that feels too big and scary to protect me.

I am afraid of a million other things.

But mostly, I'm afraid of showing my feelings. I am afraid *of* my feelings. I am buried under them. And this has caused me to stifle my humanness—which, it turns out, is 100 percent of what I am made of.

It is impossible to be me, like *this*.

What I realize next is that I have needed illness. I have needed illness because it has protected me from all the things I don't feel brave enough to say, feel, and be. It's easier to be sick than to say no when that's what I want to say. It is easier to be sick than to try to be perfect. It is easier to be sick and buried under emotions than to feel them. This is perhaps the hardest reality I've ever had to accept, because who runs around the world looking for a cure if they really don't want it?

Me.

At first, I worry that this means that being sick has been my fault. But the truth is, illness is not my fault, and even if it is, who cares anyway? Because if I want to get better, it has to be my responsibility.

Being sick does not come from failing, or from any failure on the part of those around you. It comes from being human. And sometimes, shit just goes sideways. We get cracked. But it's clear now that I'm going to have to find the glue for all my cracks. I'm going to have to learn to feel all the damn feelings when I need to feel them. And I'm going to have to learn how to let them go.

Yes.

The process of releasing all the old emotions and unhealthy patterns that have been entangled in my body becomes a journey of its own. It will not be quick, but it will become the turning point for everything I've been working toward.

I start with some of what I already know from India. *Nam myoho renge kyo. Nam myoho renge kyo. Nam myoho renge kyo.* I am chanting to bring my wise self, my inner Buddha, out. I am chanting for miracles. I also discover some new methods so that I can release stuck emotions from my body, such as the Emotional Freedom Technique, working with my chakras, and clearing unhealthy patterns from my subconscious mind (it turns out it was pretty muddy in there). I even create some of my very own tools. I do whatever I can to let everything out. What I'm doing is working. All of what I've been holding on to is falling out of me. It is sometimes painful, but it's not difficult or complicated. (P.S. I tried yoga again. Still hate it.)

After just several months, I begin to sense a sturdiness inside of me that I've never had. I am less afraid than I've ever been. I am more relaxed. I start being kinder to myself. When I make a mistake, I forget about it. When I call myself a name, I stop. When I am upset, I share it, even though showing my insides is still not easy for me to do. Maybe most important, I am getting so good at being with my feelings. I do not ignore and persist. I *listen*. And I do it without too much judgment.

I am becoming me. It's getting easier.

Yes.

My physical symptoms start to fade ever so slowly over time. My periods start to get better and I decide to keep my uterus indefinitely. My legs are strong and never tingle. I have more energy. I can eat every kind of food again without any allergies. My lab tests come back with less and less wrong and more and more right. I catch a cold and do not relapse as doctors warned I would. I am not swallowing pills or running around the world to make this happen.

And then, one day, all my lingering symptoms are healed. I am keeping this boat steady . . . for real this time! I may never be pristine and perfect, but I don't care. There is no more hiding *me*. I frequently skip wearing makeup, change my hair color and style with my mood, and allow myself to cry more easily and more often than I have ever cried in my life. I say no when I want to (at least, most of the time). Sometimes I eat too much pizza, lose complete Zen-like perspective, and forget everything I've learned. But I am healthier than ever before, because I do *being human* so much better now. In fact, I am finally not just doing it, but embracing it.

It is true what they say, that you can never go back in time and change your life. But you can always go back and heal anyway. Little by little, I found myself and I brought her back. I aligned her fully with my heart and all the ways I knew I was meant to live. I finally saw that all my struggles turned out to be more than just years of suffering; they were a metamorphosis into that which I was always meant to be.

The actual stem cells have become a smaller part of my story than I ever imagined they would be. In the end, they were not the singular cure, but the catalyst for my ultimate healing. They led me to India, where I had to struggle in ways I never had, in order to grow in ways I didn't know existed. I needed to feel alone in order to find my connection to myself and who I was in the world. I had to be misunderstood so I could learn detachment from how other people received my expression. I had to be forced away from obsessively focusing on my symptoms so I could see how life shifts as you shift your focus. Somewhere in between the time I arrived in Delhi and the time I left, I went from an existence committed to *killing* Lyme to an existence committed to *healing* me. I had to acknowledge the parts of me that were saved when I stopped fueling the war on Lyme—for I was throwing the energy of that fight into my very own body. I had to learn to squeeze my eyes shut tight, feel safe in the dark of my life, let go, and trust. And I needed to go to India to collect those words from Dr. Shroff so I had them when I needed them most. Arguably, this was just as important for me as any kind of treatment.

All of this was unseen while I was deep in the valleys of illness and despair; but when at last I found my way to the peak, and the dust of my own trek settled, the entire picture became unmistakably clear.

My beautiful, bold, life-changing adventure in India could take me only so far. The rest was always up to me.

Yes.

• • •

IT IS IN the hammering rain of October 2011 that I glide down the aisle in my white lace wedding dress. My feet are bare and my toes are painted sky blue. From the deck of this old red barn, you can see the rolling green hills of Massachusetts dotted with the radiant hues of fall— scarlet, crimson, and mustard. Mom and I cling to each other as we make our way toward David. He is standing at the front to officiate the ceremony, fulfilling the honor that Dad had planned to do. Zach is the most handsome ring bearer, and his little sister, Emma, our new niece, is the perfect flower girl.

I turn and face the crowd to see Charlotte coming toward me, escorted by her aunt Val. Charlotte's blue Converse sneakers pop out from under her dress and match the polish on my toes. Bunches of simple lavender, Janet's favorite, are wrapped in burlap for our bouquets.

Inside the barn, twinkle lights and dinner are waiting, while a henna artist paints the spirit of India onto our guests' hands and feet.

"Hey, Mama, did you miss Dad tonight?" I ask her, holding a blueberry beer in my hand. And because we are safe in each other's truth, she doesn't have to think about it.

"No," she says, with slight surprise. But I don't miss him either—I think because he is here.

When the last guests have been kissed good-bye, our family sloshes through the wide-open flooded field and out to a massive stretching tree. The moon lights the way. Under that tree, with its hovering branches and strong, solid trunk, we blow Dad's ashes from our damp hands into the air and I watch them float for a long moment.

My life feels as wide and high as the sky.

As we gallop back to safety, to warmth, and to our new version of family, I feel my feet sinking into the wet grass. My heart is beating so hard it is in my throat. My beautiful wife's hand is wrapped around mine, and the laughs of our favorite people are echoing all around us. In this moment, and in a million different ones that will come after, we will continue to remind each other that life goes on, and we do too.

In the years to come, with my bride beside me, these strong feet of mine will travel to many extraordinary places— to the blissful beaches of Mexico, back into the sacred hills of Ojai, across the roaring red sand of South Africa, and through the sun-drenched cobbled streets of Italy. Sometimes Dad will travel with us. The dust from his ashes will gently drift from a bridge over the neon Las Vegas strip, settle beneath a tree outside his favorite camera store in San Francisco, and slip through the gates of Buckingham Palace in London. One day, David, Tatiana, and Mom will carry him back to India and set him free in the holiest of all places: the Ganges. From a small boat off the banks of the river, they will participate in a traditional Hindu ceremony where the ashes of the deceased are released so their souls can be transported to heaven. But that will not be his only resting place in the land he loved so much. He will also be memorialized outside Nutech hospital on a concrete wall containing an imprint of my mom's hand and a pinch of his ashes. Mom's love of India will remain strong, bringing her back there six more times, with who knows how many more trips to come.

Little did I know that my trip would also inspire dozens of Lyme patients to follow my footsteps to Delhi. For some, the improvements would be vast. For others, there would still be much more work to do.

What I could never have imagined is that today I would be sharing with so many others what I traveled so far to learn: that you can find parts of what you need in a million different places, but you always have to come home, to yourself, for the cure.

People ask me the hardest questions I've ever had to answer. *Now that you know what you know, could you have healed without antibiotics? Without stem cells? What would you say to someone who is just starting?*

There is no perfect answer, but my truth is this.

In the end, you can't dissect your life and pick out what you could have lived without. The epically hard and beautifully brilliant moments I experienced in my search for a cure could not, for me, have unfolded in any way but exactly as they did. I didn't need any of it, but I also needed all of it. I was so comfortably uncomfortable in my life that nothing inside of me would have changed until it felt like the whole world was caving in and no one was left to save me except me. The growing and stretching and sometimes wailing into the dark black sky had to happen for me exactly as it did. It laid the sacred groundwork for the rebuilding of my soul. India was not the beginning and it was not the end. India was only the place that I collected more of the pieces.

Saving my own life was not a single act of courage nor a random act of desperation. It wasn't even, in the end, about attaining perfect physical health. It was a long, slow, burning, uncontrollable yearning to simply meet myself once again.

Sometimes you make healing happen with the strength and sheer will to survive; and sometimes you do it in the quietest moments when you feel like you are doing nothing at all. You do it by saying yes to the ugly parts of you that you wish you didn't have, reminding yourself to *let go let go let go*, harnessing your inner Ganesha when obstacles arise, telling yourself all of the truth all of the time, repeating the *I'm good enough* story when you feel otherwise, extinguishing your brain on fire, trusting that *when you know you know*, and remembering you can always get off the mat and begin again. Sometimes, if you're lucky, you'll even find some surprise inflatable chocolate cake to get you through. There will be days that you'll prevail as the hero of your own story, and nights when you'll barely scrape yourself up off the floor. But you must take it all as necessary steps and proceed.

Keep asking the questions that point to the truth of who you are. When you hear the answers, *listen*. This is how you own your story. This is how you transform who you think you should be into who you really are. This is how you become the path you've been waiting for. This is how you do it. *This* is how you save your life.

Acknowledgments

There are many people in my life who have my heart. But there are a few people without whom this book would not be the epic dream come true it is today.

My wife, Charlotte: You are the best of everything I've ever known, and by a million miles, the thing in my life that was most worth waiting for.

My family, a.k.a. the Fockers: Thank you for being the people whom I never ever want to live without. Each of you has helped me save my life in more ways than you know. Lauren and Craig: for letting me not only crash your house and your life, but for including me in every part of both. You gave me what my heart needed most. Tatiana: who traveled across states, and then the globe, to so selflessly be with me. You've been my sister from the start. David: for being the most loving and dependable dude I know. Val and Alan: the greatest and most gracious beta readers a girl could ask for. And Zach: whose perfect little squishy newborn face was always my greatest impetus for survival.

My literary agent, Steve Harris: Thank you for being the extraordinary champion of my projects, the best midday margaritas date in the world, and an all-around incredible human being. This book was always our *meant to be*, but hell if I'm letting you get away after this. We are Team 22, forever.

My two author BFFs—Sara DiVello: Endless gratitude to you for always being my rock, but especially this past year. I struck solid gold when I found you. There is #notablelikeourtable and it will forever be the very best one there is. Nadine Nettmann: Our texts and champagne breakfasts have been one of my greatest joys of being an author. Let's keep deciding to write books, crying because of them, and then convincing each other to do it all again. P.S. I think we're gonna need more champagne.

Kate Kerr-Clemenson: You've helped me to reach further than I ever could have done alone. Thank you for your never-ending genius, and even more, for your friendship.

Jay: Thank you for doing everything you did when it was so hard to do.

My doctors in India, Dr. Shroff and Dr. Ashish: I could never express my thanks for all the unexpected ways you broke my world wide open. Dr. Sudeep Sharma: Thank you for being an amazing doctor and a true friend to my family. And to all my doctors from all the years, whether you were able to help me or not, for being part of a bigger and more perfect picture than I could ever see.

My publishing family—Diana Ventimiglia: Thank you for pushing me to tell my story in the most interesting way possible, even though starting each chapter with "Picture It, Sicily, 1922" would have been both our favorite. You are the coolest editor on the whole block. Also, thank you for being a friend. Michele Martin: Your care, expertise, quick wit, and impeccable talent are truly one-of-a-kind. Thank you for saying the yes that brought this book into the world. I could not be more grateful to you. Marla Daniels: A million thank-yous for jumping into this project, head first, and with total ease. Your support in the final haul helped me to arrive in a better way than I ever could have without you. The entire team at Simon & Schuster: Thank you for your brilliant ideas and attention to detail, and for always having everything totally under control. You rock.

The people of India: My deepest gratitude goes to you, for welcoming me into your country, showering me with love, and showing me that anyplace in the world can become home.

Finally, thank you to these incredible literary superwomen, who inspire me to type my truth each time I put my fingers on the keys—Elizabeth Gilbert: for going to

India first and making me believe I could do it, maybe even gracefully. I was wrong about the grace, but you're still my hero. Glennon Doyle: for making books that remind me we can write hard things. Cheryl Strayed: for reminding me that sometimes we have to go into the wild for answers, only to realize we carried them from the start. Anne Lamott: for convincing me that even you write shitty first drafts. And for every single word in each of your books.